치과 영어 핸드북

치과종사자를 위한 영어대화의 훈련

■역 자■

정 원 균 · 정 한 성 · 김 남 희

■감 수■

Shimono Masaki

도쿄치과대학 치과위생사전문학교장, 도쿄치과대학 교수

■저 자■

Sano Satsuki

이케미도쿄치과위생사전문학교 강사, 쇼와대학의학부 부속간호전문학교 겸임강사

Sano Tsukasa

도쿄치과대학교수, 도쿄치과대학 치과위생사전문학교 정강사,
이케미도쿄치과위생사전문학교 강사, 와세다의학원 치과위생사전문학교 강사

Nakamura Nobuko

쇼와대학의학부 부속간호전문학교 겸임강사, 릿교여학원 단기대학 비상근강사

Suzanne Knowlton

쇼와대학 조교수

대한나래출판사

DaehanNarae Publishing, Inc.

Deokwon Bldg. #202
102-65 Yongdu-dong
Dongdaemun-gu
SEOUL 130-820, KOREA
TEL: +82-2-922-0840
FAX: +82-2-922-0841
E-mail: dhpub@chol.com
Website: www.dhpub.com

Title of the original Japanese language edition:
Shikayou Eigo Handbook
by Sano Satsuki et al.

ISBN 978-89-5741-102-5

Printed in Korea

감수에 부쳐

현대사회는 전 세계에 걸쳐 사람과 정보의 교류가 이루어지고 있습니다. 우리는 어디에 살든지 실시간으로 지구 곳곳의 정보를 구할 수 있습니다. 하늘의 관문이라고 하는 나리타공항은 이를 통해 드나드는 사람이 1년에 3,200만 명에 이르고, 여기에서 유통되는 돈도 무려 220만 엔 정도라고 합니다. 일본에는 이 곳 말고도 많은 공항이나 항구가 있기 때문에 이를 모두 합하면 어마어마한 숫자의 사람과 물자가 이동하고 있습니다.

외국을 여행하거나 외국에 거주하는 일본인이 크게 늘어나고 있습니다. 일본에 거주하는 외국인도 증가하여 현재 약 170만 명에 이른다고 합니다. 우리 주변에는 많은 외국인이 살고 있으며, 그 가운데 일본어를 능숙하게 구사하는 사람도 있지만 국제화시대의 공용어는 역시 영어입니다.

따라서 의료서비스 현장에서도 영어를 사용한 의사소통이 중요합니다. 치통이나 치석제거, 정기검진을 위해 치과를 찾는 외국인이 많아지고 있습니다. 이러한 외국인과 의사소통을 원활히 하기 위해서 영어가 필요한 것은 두말할 나위가 없습니다.

이 책은 접수에서 다음 약속 때까지 진료실에서 나누는 대화, 환자의 정확한 증상을 수집할 때 사용하는 표현, 방사선촬영, 약의 복용법 등 진료현장에서 일하고 있는 치과위생사에게 필요한 기초적인 실무영어를 소개하고 있습니다. 치과전문용어도 많긴 하지만 내용이 어렵지 않으며, 그림이 있어 이해하기 쉽고 동기부여에도 도움이 될 것입니다. 이 책은 장마다 어휘, 말하기, 영문법, 활용, 연습문제로 꾸며져 있어 스스로 공부하면서 진도를 나갈 수 있습니다. 독자께서 반복학습을 통해 실무영어를 몸에 익히기를 바랍니다. 이 책은 장차 치과에서 활동할 치위생(학)과 학생의 교과서로도 적당할 것으로 생각하여 감수를 하였으며, 이에 여러분께 추천 드리는 바입니다.

Shimono Masaki

머 리 말

쇼핑을 가거나 산책을 할 때 우리의 생활주변에서 영어를 어렵지 않게 접할 수 있습니다. 일본에서도 영어의 필요성이 점점 강조되고 있으며, 병원이나 치과의원도 그 예외는 아닙니다. 하지만 전문적인 치의학 영어가 늘 필요한 것은 아닙니다. 일상에서 사용하기 편한 용어로 외국인 환자와 의사소통을 할 수 있다면 그것으로 충분하다고 생각합니다.

이 책은 치위생(학)과의 학생과 임상에 근무하는 치과위생사, 치과기공사, 치과보조원 및 접수원 등의 치과종사자를 대상으로 쓴 치과진료실의 "실전" 영어책입니다. 치과종사자가 이 책을 통하여 외국인 환자가 쉽게 이해할 수 있는 기본적인 영어표현을 공부하고, 이를 실제의 임상 현장에서 활용할 수 있기를 바랍니다.

자신의 생각을 상대방에게 잘 전달하기 위해서는 많은 내용을 하나의 문장으로 길게 표현하기보다 몇 개의 짧은 문장으로 나누어 간단히 말하는 것이 좋습니다. 따라서 이 책은 〈짧은 문장의 간단한 표현〉과 〈최소한의 단어를 이용한 표현〉이라는 기본원칙에 따라 집필하였습니다.

이 책의 본문은 "어휘(Vocabulary)"와 "핵심문장(Key sentences)"을 먼저 공부한 후에 "말하기(Speaking)와 영문법(Grammar)" 항목에서 이를 직접 연습하고, "활용(Practice)" 에서 연습문제를 풀도록 꾸몄습니다. 각 장에는 "초점(Focus)" 항목을 두어 본문에서 다룬 문법이나 관련내용을 정리하고, "연습문제(Exercise)"에서 다시 한 번 복습할 수 있도록 하였습니다.

불안하고 두려운 마음으로 치과를 찾는 외국 환자에게는 치과종사자와 의사소통이 매우 중요합니다. 이 책이 이러한 역할에 작은 도움이 되기를 바랍니다.

저자대표 **Sano Satsuki**

역자 서문

이 역서는 일본의 도쿄치과대학과 몇몇 치과위생사전문학교에서 치과위생사 교육을 담당하고 있는 교수들이 저술하신 '치과용 영어 핸드북(2006년)' 이란 제목의 원서를 우리말로 옮긴 것입니다.

우리 사회와 대학에 국제화나 세계화라는 가치가 보편화된 것은 어제 오늘의 일이 아니며, 그 중심에 영어를 사용한 의사소통의 문제가 있습니다. 이러한 흐름은 의료시장의 개방을 눈앞에 두고 있는 우리나라의 보건의료 부분도 예외가 아닙니다. 우리 치위생계나 치과계도 이에 대한 구체적인 준비를 해나가야 할 것입니다.

치과진료실에서 외국인 환자를 만나는 일이 이제는 특별하지 않게 되었습니다. 말이 통하지 않는 것만큼 대인관계에서 겁나는 일은 없습니다. 하지만 치과위생사를 포함한 치과종사자들이 쉽고 간단한 영어로 외국인 환자와 의사소통을 할 수 있다면 그것 이상으로 더 어렵고 복잡한 영어회화가 필요할까 싶습니다.

제가 처음 이 책을 접하고 받은 느낌은 그 내용이 매우 간결하고 쉽다는 점입니다. 따라서 이 책이 실무영어의 교육에 많은 시간과 노력을 할애하기 어려운 우리나라 대학의 치위생(학)과 교육여건에 적합하다고 생각하였습니다. 책의 분량도 부담이 없으며, 치과진료실에서 바로 적용할 수 있는 구체적인 영어대화의 용례를 압축하여 담고 있습니다. 아울러 이 책은 치과의사와 치과기공사, 접수원 등에게도 도움이 될 것으로 판단하였습니다.

이 역서를 펴내게 된 직접적인 계기는 연세대학교 치과대학의 정한성 교수의 조언 때문이었습니다. 평소 치과위생사 교육에 많은 관심과 애정을 보내 주신 정한성 교수께서 일본 현지에서 이 책을 직접 소개해 주셨고, 우리말로 출간할 수 있도록 여러모로 도움을 주셨습니다. 아울러 이 책의 교정 작업을 도와주신 연세대학교 원주의과대학 치위생학과의 한선영, 김아름, 정혜령, 최진아 조교 선생님께도 감사를 드립니다.

2007년의 끝자락에서

역자대표 **정 원 균**

차 례

UNIT 1 I'm a dental hygienist.

Vocabulary

① 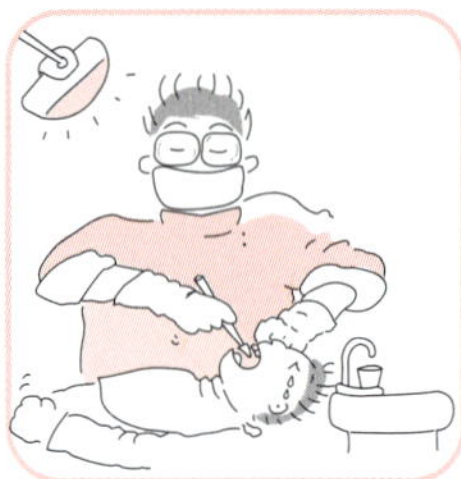
dentist

② 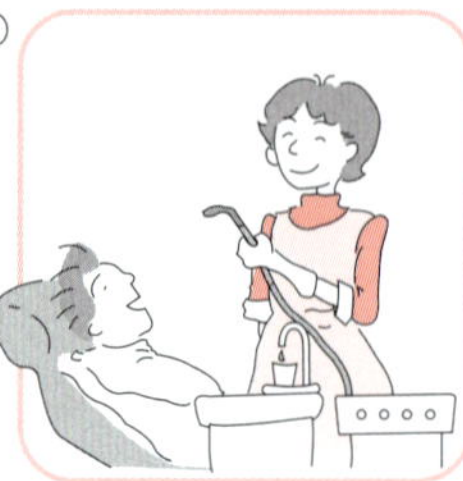
dental hygienist

③ 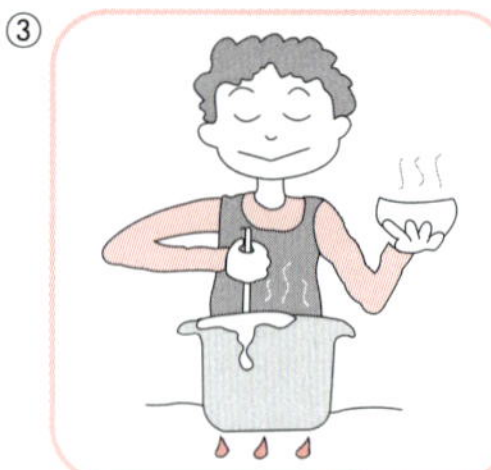
housewife

④ 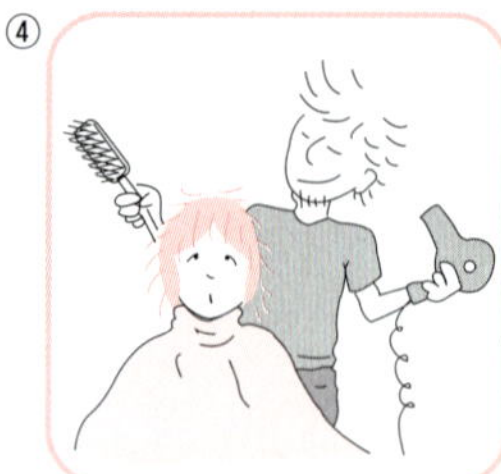
hairdresser

⑤ 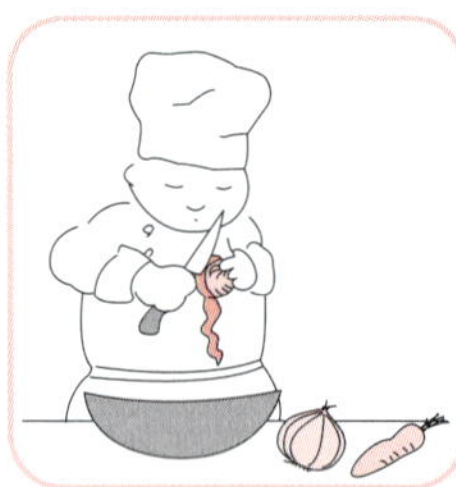
cook

⑥ 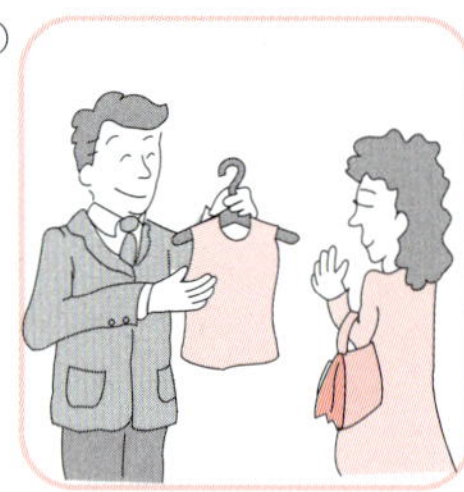
salesperson

⑦ 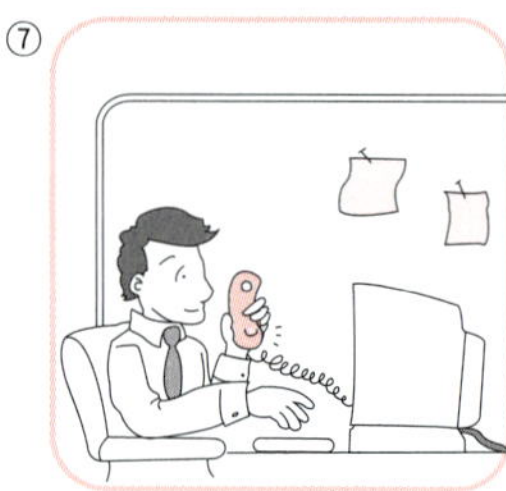
office worker

⑧ 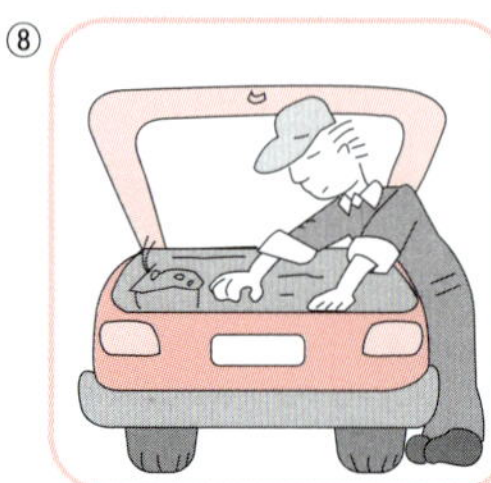
mechanic

① 치과의사 ② 치과위생사 ③ 주부 ④ 미용사 ⑤ 요리사 ⑥ 판매원 ⑦ 회사원 ⑧ 정비사

☞ 치과조무사: dental assistant 치과기공사: dental technician

Speaking & Grammar

① My name is Young-sook Lee.
② I'm from Seoul.
③ I'm not a student.
④ I'm a dental hygienist.
⑤ I'm single.

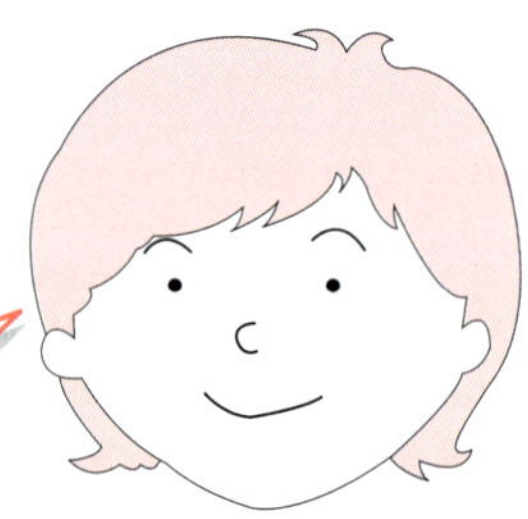

⑥ My parents are in Wonju.
⑦ They're office workers.

⑧ My sister is married.
⑨ She's a housewife.

☞ I'm = I am from:··· 출신 They're = They are She's = She is
single : 독신 ⇔ married : 결혼한 parent : 부모 (아버지와 어머니) in : ··· (안)에

① 제 이름은 이영숙입니다. ② 저는 서울 출신입니다. ③ 저는 학생이 아닙니다. ④ 저는 치과위생사입니다.
⑤ 저는 독신입니다. ⑥ 저의 부모님은 원주에 사십니다. ⑦ 저의 부모님은 회사원이십니다. ⑧ 언니는 결혼했습니다.
⑨ 언니는 주부입니다.

1. 위의 예를 참고하여 영어로 표현해 보세요.

My name is ···	My boy friend is ··· in ···	I'm from ···
He's from ···	I'm not ···	He's a ···
I'm a ···	He's not ···	I'm ···

2. 친구와 역할을 나누어 서로 영어로 질문해 보세요.

① Are you a dental hygienist?	Yes, I am. / No, I'm not.
a housewife?	
an office worker?	
a salesperson?	
a dental assistant?	
② Where are you from?	I'm from…
③ How old are you?	25 (years old).
④ How are your parents?	They are fine.
⑤ Is your mother busy?	Yes, she is. / No, she isn't.
⑥ Is your father tall or short?	He's short.
⑦ Is your sister single or married?	She's single.
⑧ What's your first (last) name?	Young-sook (Lee).
⑨ What's your occupation?	I'm a dental hygienist.
⑩ What's your nationality?	I'm Korean.
⑪ What's your e-mail address?	gogo12@dot.com.
⑫ What's your cellphone number?	090-8889-6760.

☞ what's = what is

① 당신은 치과위생사이세요? ② 어디 출신이세요? 나이가 어떻게 되세요? ④ 부모님은 어떠신가요?
⑤ 어머님은 바쁘신가요? ⑥ 아버님은 키가 크신가요 아니면 작으신가요?
⑦ 언니(또는 동생)는 독신인가요 아니면 결혼하셨나요? ⑧ 성함이 어떻게 되시죠? ⑨ 어떤 직업에 종사하세요?
⑩ 당신의 국적은 어디세요?(당신은 어느 나라 사람이세요?) ⑪ 이메일 주소가 어떻게 되시나요? ⑫ 휴대전화 번호가 어떻게 되시지요?

Practice

3. 빈 칸을 채워 문장을 완성하세요.

① ( ) you a dental hygienist?

② What ( ) your son's name?

③ Rita's teeth ( ) white.

④ My children ( ) in the UK.

⑤ Jim and I are classmates. ( ) are good friends.

⑥ Julia and Tom are from the USA. ( ) are American.

⑦ Where are you and Miki? ( ) are at home.

☞ son : 아들 teeth : tooth(치아)의 복수형 children : child(자녀)의 복수형
the UK : 영국 the USA : 미국 at home : 집에 있는

4. (　　)의 단어를 사용하여 의문문을 만드세요.

① (she / a student) ⇒ Is she a student?

② (your boy friend / short)

③ (you / from / where)

④ (your / what / phone number)

⑤ (you / married)

⑥ (your / bag / where)

5. 국가에 맞는 국적을 빈 칸에 쓰세요.

~~Japanese~~	Chinese	Brazilian	American	French	Spanish	Irish
German	Russian	British	Greek	Indian	Korean	Turkish

Country		Nationality	Country		Nationality
Japan	일본	Japanese	The UK	영국	________
The USA	미국	________	Spain	스페인	________
China	중국	________	Turkey	터키	________
Germany	독일	________	Greece	그리스	________
Russia	러시아	________	France	프랑스	________
Brazil	브라질	________	India	인도	________
Ireland	아일랜드	________	Korea	대한민국	________

6. 옳게 쓴 표현에 밑줄을 그으세요.

① Are you from Japan / Japanese ?

② Is she China / Chinese ?

③ Are they from Greek / Greece ?

④ Are you German / Germany ?

⑤ Is he India / Indian ?

⑥ Are they from Spanish / Spain ?

7. 다음의 대답을 이끌어낼 수 있는 질문을 만들어 보세요.

① A : ______________________ B : I'm British.

② A : ______________________ B : I'm from the UK.

③ A : ______________________ B : 03-2435-6797.

④ A : ______________________ B : I'm a salesperson.

⑤ A : ______________________ B : 123, Sindang 2-dong, Jung-gu

⑥ A : ______________________ B : I'm single.

Answer Key

3

① Are ② is ③ are ④ are ⑤ We ⑥ They ⑦ We

4

② Is your boy friend short ? ③ Where are you from ?
④ What is your phone number ? ⑤ Are you married ?
⑥ Where is your bag ?

5

The USA– American China– Chinese Germany– German Russia– Russian
Brazil– Brazilian Ireland–Irish The UK – British Spain–Spanish
Turkey–Turkish Greece–Greek France–French India–Indian Korea–Korean

6

② Chinese ③ Greece ④ German ⑤ Indian ⑥ Spain

7

① What's your nationality ? ② Where are you from ?
③ What's your telephone number ? ④ What's your occupation ?
⑤ What's your address ? ⑥ Are you single or married ?

UNIT 1 FOCUS

《am, is, are의 사용》

영어의 인칭은 〈나〉 〈당신〉 〈그 밖의 사람〉의 세 가지입니다. 또 그 각각에는 「단수(하나)」와 「복수(둘 이상)」가 있습니다. 이를 잘 기억하세요.

	(하나)			(둘 이상)		
(나)	I	**am**	a student.	We	**are**	dental hygienists.
(당신)	You	**are**	tall.	You	**are**	kind.
(그 밖의 사람)	She/He/It	**is**	from China.	They	**are**	from Brazil.

《부정과 의문》

is, am, are를 사용한 문장에 「~가 아니다」라는 부정을 표현하려면 am, is, are에 not을 연결합니다. 의문문일 때에는 am, is, are가 문장의 제일 앞에 옵니다.

〈부정〉

I	am	**not**	a student.
He (She/ It)	is	**not**	tall.
We (You/ They)	are	**not**	from China.

〈의문〉

Are	you		a student? tall?
Is	he (she/ it)		from China?
Are	they (we/ you)		

〈대답〉

Yes, I am. No, I'm not.
Yes, he is. No, he isn't.
Yes, they are. No, they aren't.

Exercise

1. 지도에 표시된 국가의 이름을 표의 빈 칸에 쓰세요.

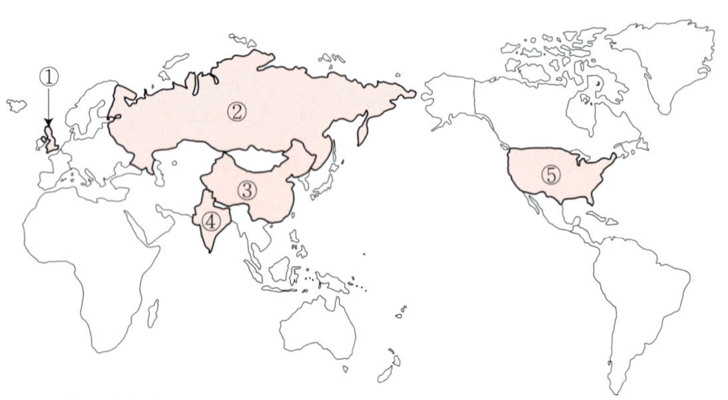

①
②
③
④
⑤

2. (1)~(5)는 사람을 설명하는 내용입니다. 이 글을 잘 읽고 student, tall, married, from Russia에 해당되는 사람의 이름은 아래 동그라미 속에, 해당되지 않는 사람의 이름은 동그라미 밖에 표시하세요. 그리고 A~H의 문장을 완성하세요.

(1) Tom is a student. He is tall. He is not married. He is from the U.S.A.

(2) Jean is a cook. He is not tall. He is married. He is from France.

(3) Mika is a student. She is not tall. She is not married. She is from Japan.

(4) Bob is a dentist. He is tall. He is not married. He is from Ireland.

(5) Natasha is a dental hygienist. She is tall. She is married. She is from Russia.

job

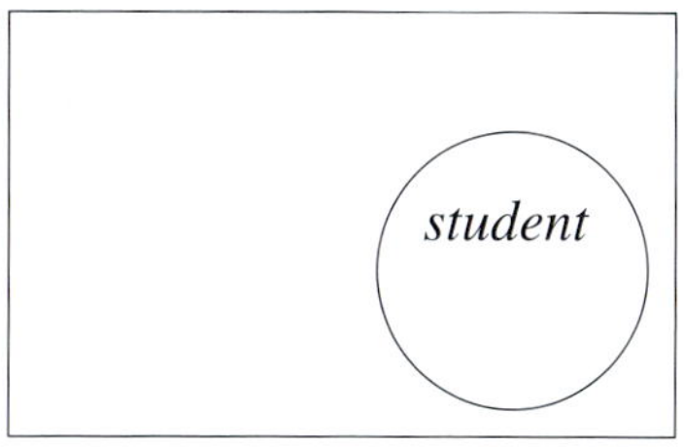

tall

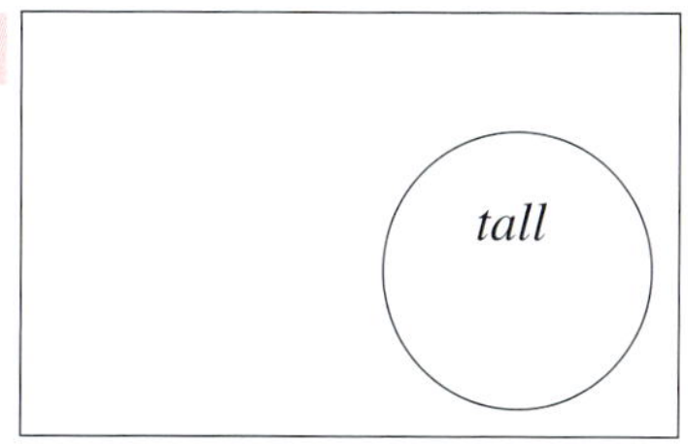

A.______________________ students.

B.______________________ not students.

C.______________________ tall.

D.______________________ not tall.

married

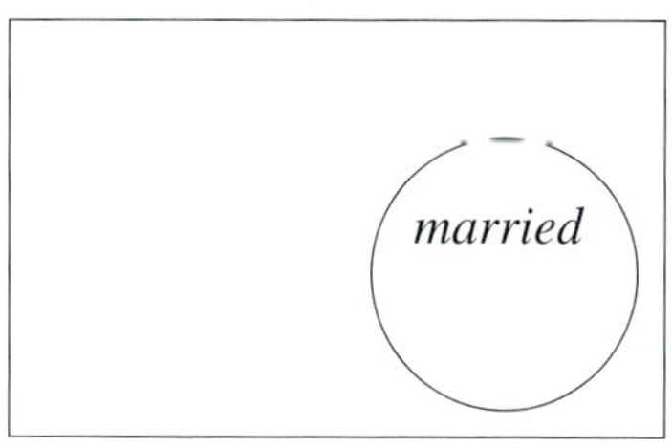

from

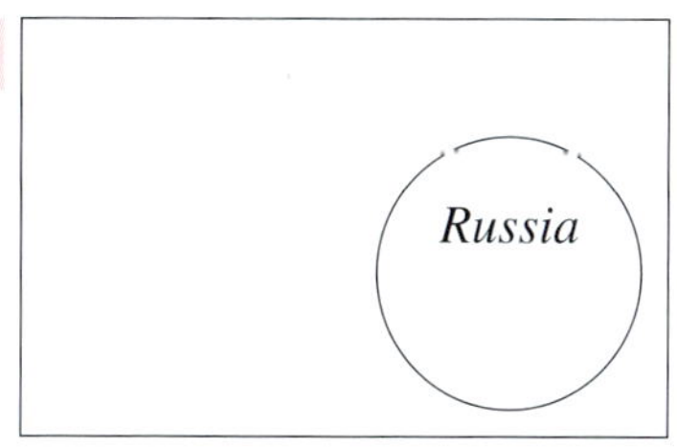

E.______________________ married.

F.______________________ not married.

G.______________________ from Russia.

H.______________________ not from Russia.

Answer Key

1 ① 영국 ② 러시아 ③ 중국 ④ 인도 ⑤ 미국

2

job	A. Tom and Mika are students.
	B. Jean, Bob and Natasha are not students.
tall	C. Tom, Bob and Natasha are tall.
	D. Jean and Mika are not tall.
married	E. Jean and Natasha are married.
	F. Tom, Mika and Bob are not married.
from Russia	G. Natasha is from Russia.
	H. Tom, jean, Mika and Bob are not from Russia.

UNIT 2 I brush my teeth.

Vocabulary

①
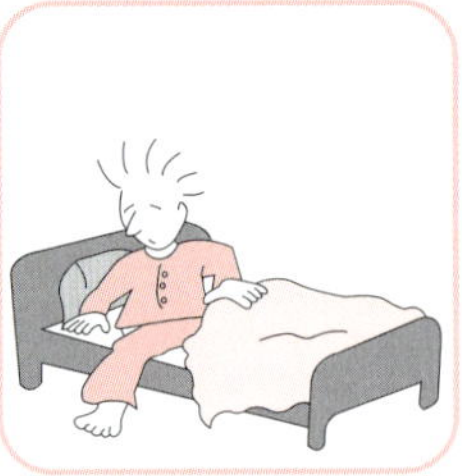
get up

②
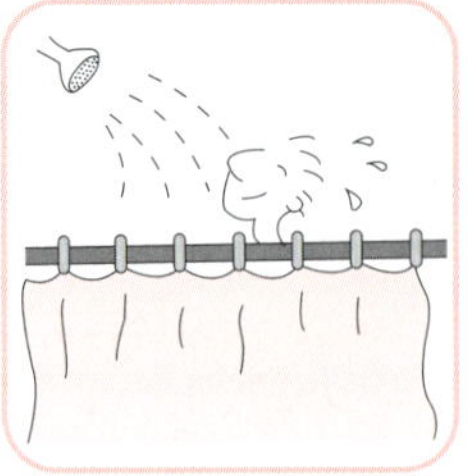
take a shower

③
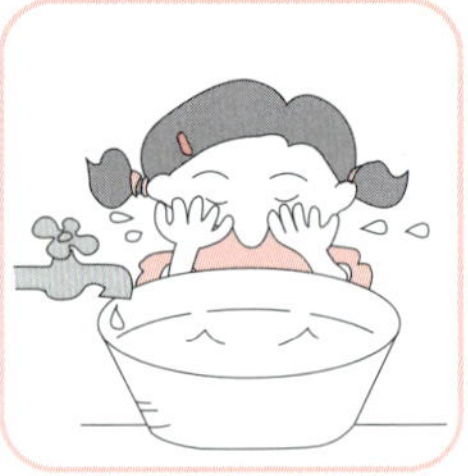
wash my face

④
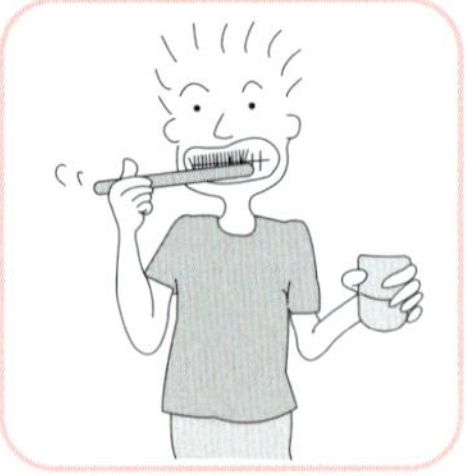
brush my teeth

⑤
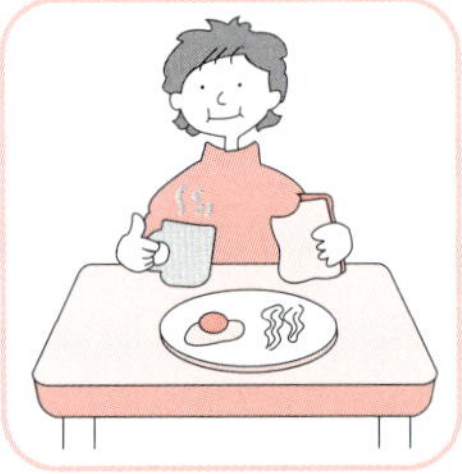
have breakfast

⑥
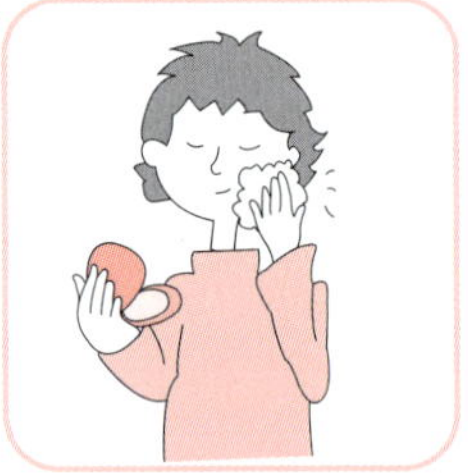
put on my makeup

⑦
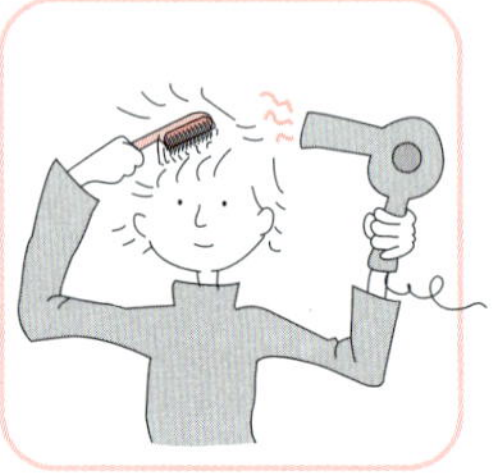
do my hair

⑧
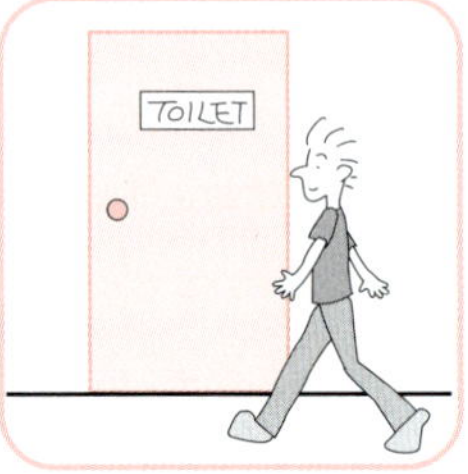

use the washroom

⑨
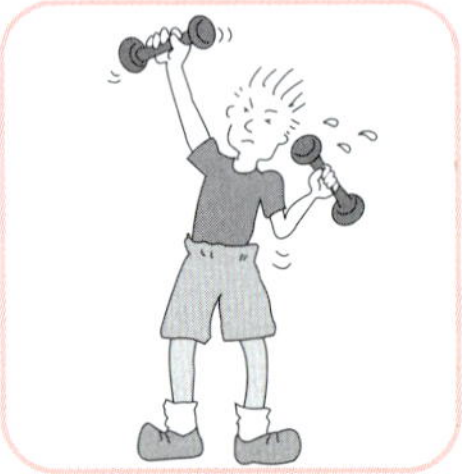
exercise

⑩
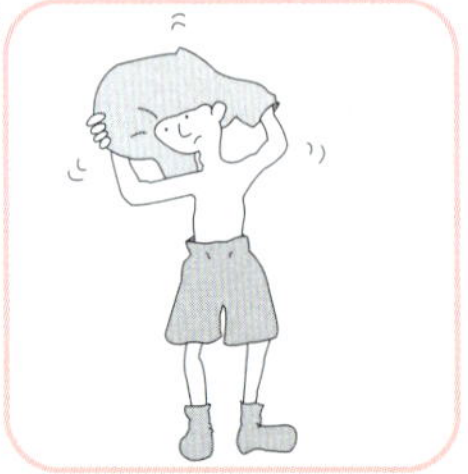
take off my clothes

⑪
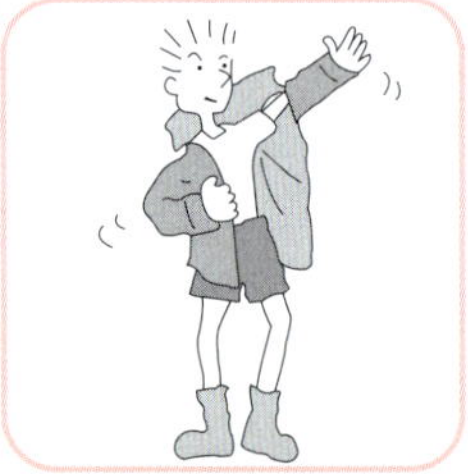
put on my clothes

⑫
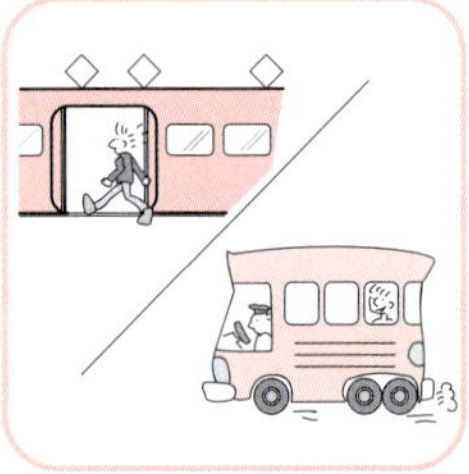
take the train/bus

① 잠에서 일어나다. ② 목욕하다. ③ 세수하다. ④ 이를 닦다. ⑤ 아침식사를 하다. ⑥ 화장을 하다. ⑦ 머리를 빗다.
⑧ 화장실에 가다. ⑨ 운동을 하다. ⑩ 옷을 벗다. 신발을 벗다. ⑪ 옷을 입다. 신발을 신다. ⑫ 지하철이나 버스를 타다.

1. 당신이 아침마다 하는 일과 하지 않는 일을 적어 보세요.

〔do〕

I get up at six thirty.

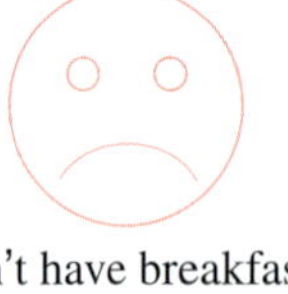
〔do not〕

I don't have breakfast.

Speaking & Grammar

2. 역할을 나누어 상대에게 서로 질문해 보세요.

① Do you have breakfast every morning?	Yes, I do. / No, I don't.
② Do you take a bath in the morning?	
③ Do you exercise every day?	
④ Do you brush your teeth after meals?	
⑤ Do you take the train?	
⑥ What do you do?	ex. I'm a dental hygienist.
⑦ Where do you live?	In Tokyo.
⑧ How do you go to school?	By bus.
⑨ When do you brush your teeth?	After meals.
⑩ What time do you go to sleep?	At about 12 p.m.
⑪ What kind of food do you like?	I like Italian food.
⑫ Where do your parents live?	In Hawaii.
⑬ What does your father do?	He is a cook.
⑭ Where does he work?	He works at a restaurant.

☞ ① 매일 아침식사를 하세요? ② 아침에 목욕을 하십니까? ③ 날마다 운동을 하세요? ④ 식사 후에는 이를 닦습니까?
⑤ 지하철을 이용하십니까? ⑥ 어떤 일을 하세요? ⑦ 어디에 사시나요? ⑧ 어떻게 통학을 하세요?
⑨ 이를 언제 닦으시나요? ⑩ 몇 시에 주무시나요? ⑪ 어떤 음식을 좋아하나요? ⑫ 부모님은 어디에 사시나요?
⑬ 아버님은 무슨 일은 하시나요? ⑭ 아버님은 어디에서 일하시는지요?

3. 영어로 질문해 보세요. 짝을 지어 Emily(A)와 Tom(B)의 역할을 각각 정합니다. 각자의 정보를 보고 A가 B에게 질문을 하면 B가 대답하고, B가 A에게 질문을 하면 A는 대답합니다.

〈Emily〉	〈A가 알고 있는 내용〉	〈B에게 하는 질문〉
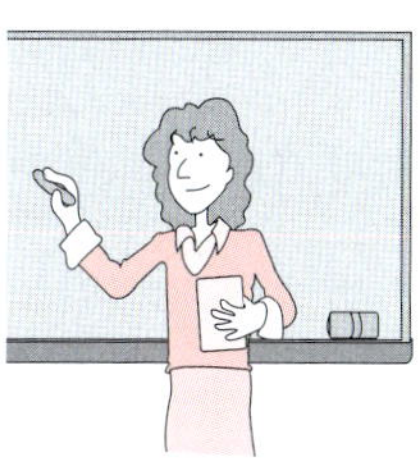	Emily is a nurse.	What does he do?
	She is American.	What ______ ?
	She is from Chicago.	Where ______ ?
	She lives in Tokyo.	Where ______ ?
	She works at a hospital.	Where ______ ?
	She goes to work by bicycle.	How ______ ?
	She likes Chinese food.	What kind of ______ ?

〈Tom〉	〈B가 알고 있는 내용〉	〈A에게 하는 질문〉
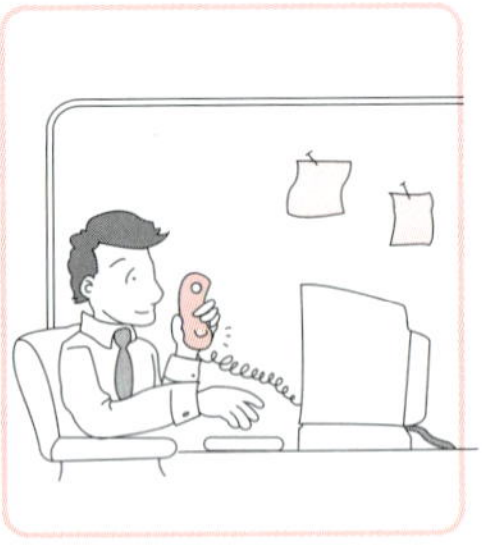	Tom is Canadian.	What is her nationality ?
	He is from Vancouver.	______________________ ?
	He is an office worker.	______________________ ?
	He lives in Seoul.	______________________ ?
	He works at a bank.	______________________ ?
	He goes to work by train.	______________________ ?
	He likes Japanese food.	______________________ ?

Practice

4. 잘못된 부분을 바르게 고치세요.

① She live in Seoul.

② Naomi don't have a sister.

③ He is speaks English.

④ My mother don't work at a bank.

⑤ Tom and Mami are goes at home.

⑥ She is eats lunch.

5. 빈 칸을 채워 질문을 완성하세요.

① ________ you speak English?	Yes, I do.
② Where ________ she from?	She is from Seoul.
③ ________ do you live?	In Tokyo.
④ ________ do you do?	I'm a dental hygienist.
⑤ ________ do you work?	I work at a dental clinic.
⑥ ________ you have any sisters or brothers?	Yes, I have a sister.
⑦ What ________ your sister do?	She is an office worker.
⑧ Where does she live?	She ________ in Seoul.
⑨ What kind of ________ do you like?	I like Italian food.
⑩ What kind of ________ does she like?	She likes popular music.

6. 빈 칸에 단어를 넣어 문장을 완성하세요.

① Are ____?

② Do ____?

③ Does ____?

④ What ____?

⑤ Where ____?

⑥ What time ____?

Answer Key

4 밑줄 친 부분은 바르게 고친 표현

① She lives in Seoul. ② Naomi doesn't have a sister.

③ He speaks English.

④ My mother doesn't work at a bank.

⑤ Tom and Mami are at home. (Tom and Mami go home.)

⑥ She eats lunch.

5

① Do ② is ③ Where ④ What ⑤ Where

⑥ Do ⑦ does ⑧ lives ⑨ food ⑩ music

UNIT 2 FOCUS

《he/she/it에는 s를 붙인다.》

「나」와 「당신」 이외에 단수의 사물이 주어일 때(he/she/it)에는 동사의 끝에 "s"를 붙입니다. 동사가 -o, -ch, -ss, -sh로 끝나면 "-es"를 붙입니다.

I (You) (We/ You/ They)	live	in Seoul.
He (She/ It)	lives	in Seoul.

I (You) (We/ You/ They)	go watch kiss wash	to Jeju. movies. Mary. shirts.
He (She/ It)	go**es** watch**es** kiss**es** wash**es**	to Jeju. movies. Mary. shirts.

《부정과 의문》

동사가 있고 「~가 아니다」라는 부정문을 만들 때에는 주어 뒤에 do not을 붙입니다. 다만, 주어가 he/she/it일 때에는 do에 "-es"를 붙여 "does not"를 씁니다. 이 때 "does"는 문장의 한 곳에만 사용하므로 동사에는 아무 것도 붙이지 않습니다. 의문문일 때는 do가 문장의 제일 앞에 옵니다.

〈부정〉

I (You) (We/You/They)	**do**	not	live in Suwon.
He (She/ It)	**does**	not	live in Suwon.

× He lives not in Suwon.

× He do not lives in Suwon.

× He does not lives in Suwon.

〈의문〉

Do	you (I) (we/ you/ they)		live in Suwon?
Does (she/ it)	he		live in Suwon?

〈대답〉

Yes, I do. No, I don't.
Yes, he does. No, he doesn't.

Exercise

1. 일상생활에서 자신의 행동을 영어로 표현해 보세요.

①
②
③
④
⑤
⑥
⑦
⑧
⑨
⑩

2. 역할을 나누어 평상시 상대의 행동에 대해 질문해 보세요. 대답을 듣고 상대방이 보통 때 무엇을 하는지 아래 표에 써 보세요.

①
②
③
④
⑤
⑥
⑦
⑧
⑨
⑩

질문을 할 때 다음의 표현을 참고하세요.

Do you...... ?　What...... ?　Where...... ?　Who...... ?
When...... ?

UNIT 3 The filling came out this morning.

Vocabulary

①
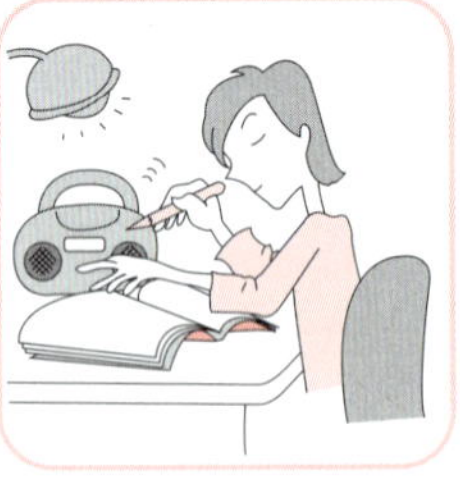
study English
(　　　　　　)

②
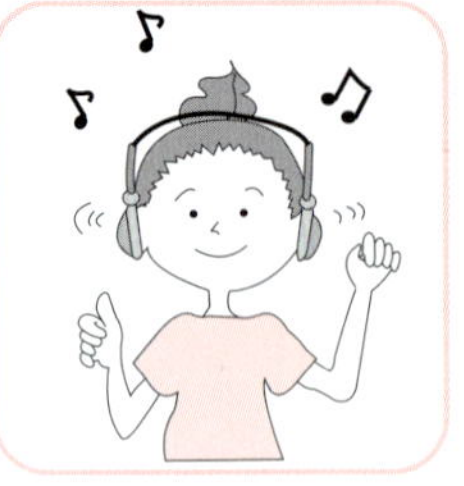
listen to music
(　　　　　　)

③
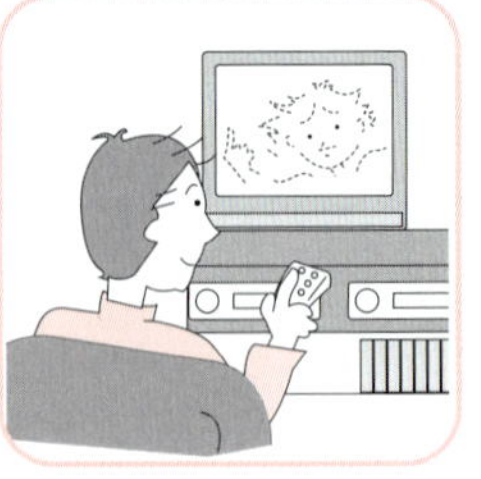
watch TV
(　　　　　　)

④
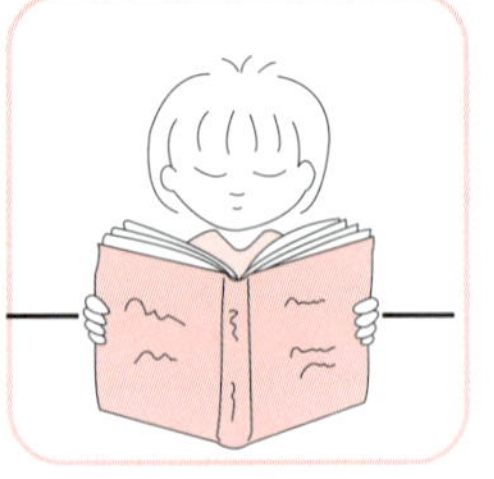
read a book
(　　　　　　)

⑤
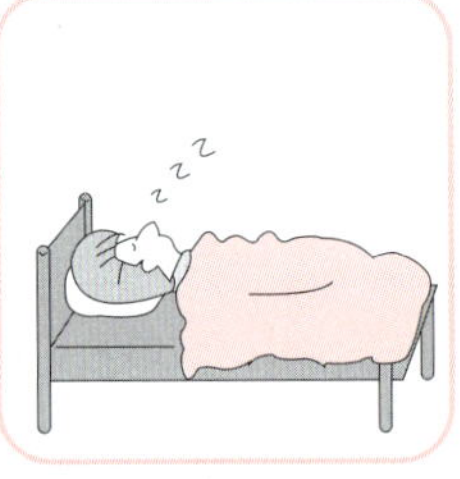
sleep
(　　　　　　)

⑥
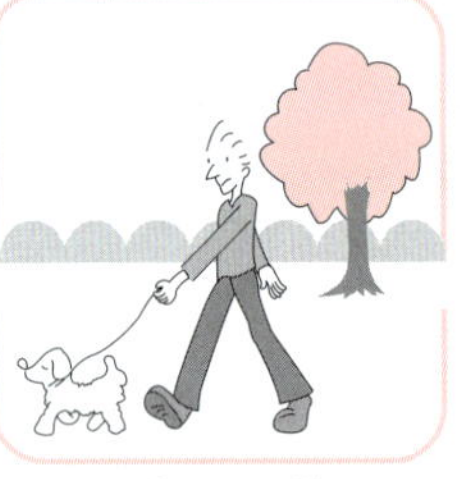
take a walk
(　　　　　　)

⑦
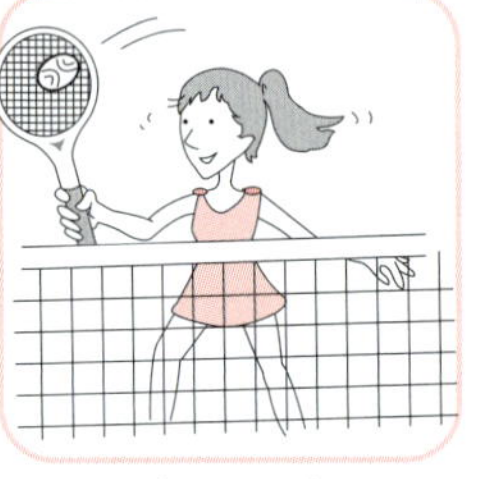
play tennis
(　　　　　　)

⑧
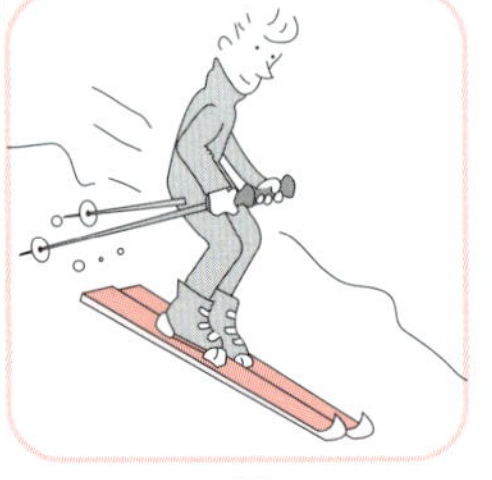
ski
(　　　　　　)

⑨
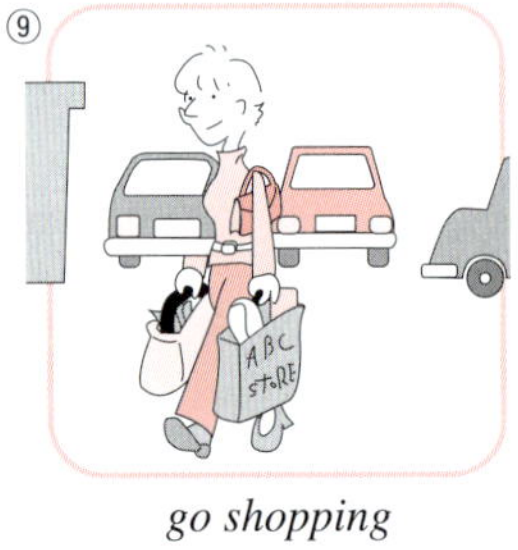

go shopping
(　　　　　　)

⑩
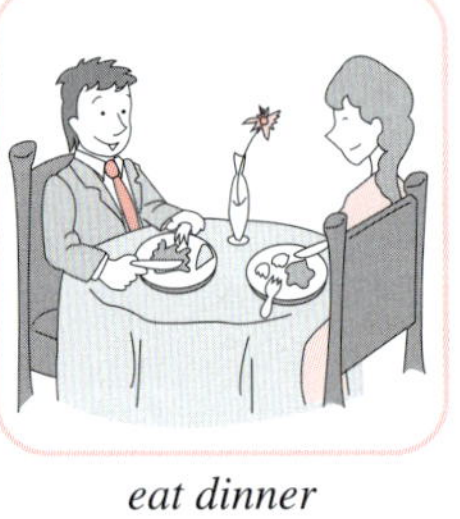
eat dinner
(　　　　　　)

⑪
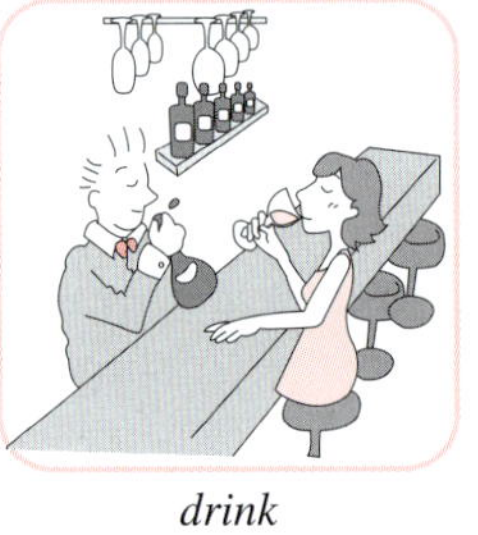
drink
(　　　　　　)

⑫
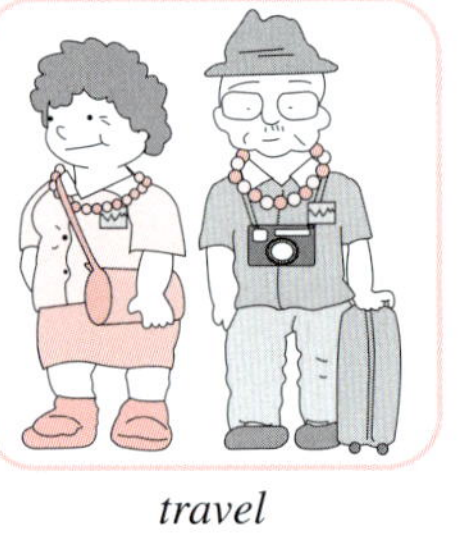
travel
(　　　　　　)

① 영어공부를 한다. ② 음악을 듣는다. ③ 텔레비전을 본다. ④ 책을 읽는다. ⑤ 잠을 잔다. ⑥ 산책을 한다. ⑦ 테니스를 친다. ⑧ 스키를 탄다. ⑨ 쇼핑을 한다. ⑩ 저녁식사를 한다. ⑪ 술을 마신다. ⑫ 여행을 간다.

1. Vocabulary의 그림 아래의 빈 칸에 동사의 과거형을 적어 보세요.

2. 주말에 한 일과 하지 않은 일을 목록으로 만들어 보세요.

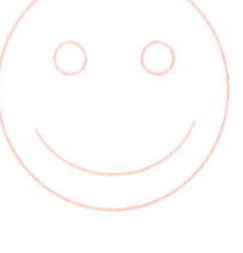

〔did〕

I studied English last weekend.

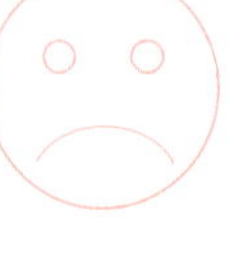

〔did not〕

I didn’t watch TV last weekend.

Speaking & Grammar

3. 역할을 나누어 상대에게 질문을 해 보세요.

① Did you watch TV yesterday?	Yes, I did. / No, I didn't.
② Did you study English yesterday?	
③ Did you go shopping last weekend?	
④ Did you read a book last week?	
⑤ Did you ski last year?	
⑥ Did you travel last year?	
⑦ What did you do last night?	e.g. I studied math.
⑧ Where did you go last weekend?	I went to Busan.
⑨ How did you come to school this morning?	By bus.
⑩ When did you take a bath yesterday?	Before dinner.
⑪ What time did you go to sleep last night?	At 11 p.m.
⑫ What kind of movies did you watch last year?	Action movies.

☞ ① 어제 텔레비전을 보셨어요? ② 어제 영어공부를 했습니까? ③ 지난 주말에 쇼핑을 하셨나요? ④ 지난주에 책을 읽었나요?
⑤ 작년에 스키를 탔습니까? ⑥ 작년에 여행을 하셨나요? ⑦ 어제 밤에 무슨 일을 했습니까? ⑧ 지난 주말에 어디를 다녀오셨나요?
⑨ 오늘 아침에 학교에 어떻게 왔습니까? ⑩ 어제 언제 목욕을 했습니까? ⑪ 어제 밤에 몇 시에 잤습니까?
⑫ 작년에 어떤 종류의 영화를 보았습니까?

4. 다음은 Steve의 현재(A)와 과거(B)에 관한 이야기입니다.
1) 동작을 표현하는 단어에 밑줄을 긋고, 동사의 현재형과 과거형을 확인해 보세요.
2) 역할을 나누어 상대에게 내용에 대한 질문을 해 보세요.

A

Steve is 55 years old. He is a dentist. He lives alone in New York. He works from Monday to Friday. He goes to his cottage in New Jersey every weekend. He doesn't watch TV or read a newspaper there. He takes a walk for many hours and watches birds. He enjoys city life and country life.

B

Steve was born in Atlanta, Georgia. He lived there with his mother, father and two brothers. He didn't study very well. When he was eighteen years old, he started work on a farm. He worked every day. After ten years, he wanted to study again and entered a university in New York. He became a dentist in 1985.

Q1 How old is Steve?

A1 ______________________________.

Q2 What is his occupation?

A2 ______________________________.

Q3 Where does he live?

A3 ______________________________.

Q4 Where does he go every weekend?

A4 ______________________________.

Q5 What does he do in New Jersey?

A5 ______________________________.

Q1 Where was Steve born?

A1 ______________________________.

Q2 How many brothers did he have?

A2 ______________________________.

Q3 What was his occupation?

A3 ______________________________.

Q4 How old was he when he entered the university?

A4 ______________________________.

Q5 When did he become a dentist?

A5 ______________________________.

Practice

5. 잘못된 부분을 바르게 고치세요.

① She playsed the piano last night.

② I goed to Daegu last week.

③ Tom studyed math this morning.

④ Emily doesn't took a bath yesterday.

⑤ My parents was angry yesterday.

⑥ She didn't took a walk in the morning.

6. 네모안의 동사를 과거형으로 고쳐 빈 칸에 써 보세요.

make	give	leave	meet	buy	write

① I (　　　　) a letter to my sister.

② He (　　　　) home at 7 : 00 this morning.

③ My father (　　　　) a shirt in the shop.

④ I (　　　　) my friend in a cafe.

⑤ Sue (　　　　) me a present.

⑥ My mother (　　　　) apple pie for me.

7. 빈 칸에 알맞은 단어를 넣고, (   )안의 단어를 적절히 고쳐 회화 문장을 완성하세요.

① A : What happened?

B : The filling (come   ) out.

☞ filling : 충전물

A : (   ) (   ) it happen?

B : This morning.

② A : Are you all right?

B : No. I (fight   ) on my way home.

A : (   ) (   ) you fight?

B : Because he (kick   ) me.

A : (   ) you hurt yourself?

B : Yes, I did. I (lose   ) my tooth.

A : (   ) you go to the dentist?

B : No, I didn't.

Answer Key

5 밑줄 친 부분은 바르게 고친 표현

① She <u>played</u> the piano last night.

② I <u>went</u> to Daegu last week.

③ Tom <u>studied</u> math this morning

④ Emily <u>didn't</u> take a bath yesterday.

⑤ My parents <u>were</u> angry yesterday.

⑥ She didn't <u>take</u> a walk in the morning.

6 ① wrote ② left ③ bought ④ met ⑤ gave ⑥ made

7 ① came, When, did ② fought, Why, did, kicked, Did, lost, Did

FOCUS

《과거형①》

동사의 과거형은 단어마다 정해져 있습니다. 동사의 규칙적인 과거형은 -ed를 붙입니다. 불규칙한 과거형은 단어에 따라 다릅니다. 이는 영어사전을 찾아 확인해 보세요. 현재형은 he/she/it이 주어일 때에는 동사에 s를 붙이며, 과거형은 주어에 관계없이 모두 같습니다.

〈규칙형〉

(i) - ed	I (You/ He /She / It) (We/ You/ They)	watch**ed** brush**ed** wash**ed**	TV. my teeth. dishes.
(ii) - d		live**d**	in Seoul.
(iii) - ied		stud**ied**	English.

〈불규칙형〉

I (You/He/She/It) (We/You/They)	**made** **went** **cut**	cookies. to Seoul. my finger.

《과거형②》

(나)	I	**was**	a student.
(당신)	You	**were**	hungry.
(그 밖의 사람)	She/He/It	**was**	angry.

We	**were**	dental hygienists.
You	**were**	married.
They	**were**	bored.

《부정과 의문》

동사가 있을 때 「~이 아니다」라는 부정문은 주어 뒤에 did not을 붙입니다. 과거형은 본문의 한 곳에만 표시하므로 동사는 과거형을 쓰지 않습니다.

〈부정〉

I (You/He/She/It) (We/You/They)	**did not** **did not** **did not**	brush my teeth. live in Jeonju. go to Gwangju.

× He lived not in Jeonju. × He did not went to Gwangju.

의문문에는 did를 문장의 제일 앞에 붙입니다. was/were가 있을 때에도 문장의 제일 앞에 씁니다.

〈의문〉

Did	I (You/He/She/It) (We/You/They)		live in Jeonju?
Was	she (he/it)		a student?
Were	they (we/you)		students?

〈대답〉

Yes, I did. No, I didn't.
Yes, she was. No, she wasn't.
Yes, they were. No, they weren't.

Exercise

1. 과거 시제를 표현하는 방법을 기억하세요.

오늘	today
어제	yesterday
그저께	the day before yesterday
사흘 전	three days ago
지난 주	last week
삼주 전	three weeks ago
지난 달	last month
다섯 달 전	five months ago
지난 해(작년)	last year
오년 전	five years ago

과거 시제를 표현하는 방법으로 「~했을 때」, 「~하기 전에」 등의 표현을 쓸 수도 있습니다.

당신이 고등학생일 적에	when you were a high school student
당신이 여기 오기 전에	before you came here

2. 역할을 나누어 상대에게 과거 시제로 질문해 보세요.

What ____________________________ this morning?

How ____________________________ this morning?

What ____________________________ yesterday?

Where ____________________________ yesterday?

Who ____________________________ yesterday?

What ____________________________ last week?

Where ____________________________ last month?

Where ____________________________ last year?

What ____________________________ when you were a high school student?

How ____________________________ when you were a high school student?

Who ____________________________ when you were a high school student?

UNIT 4 May I have your name?

Key sentences

Is this your first visit? (처음 오셨습니까? [초진이세요?])

Yes, it is. (네, 그렇습니다.)

Do you have an insurance card?
(건강보험증이 있으십니까?)

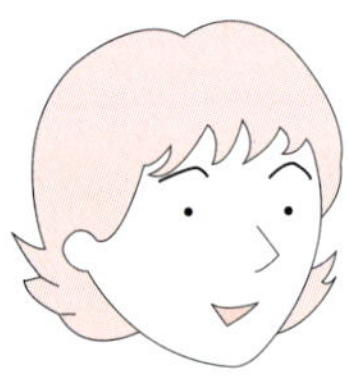

Yes, I do. (네, 있습니다.)

May I ask you some questions?
(질문 몇 가지 드려도 될까요?)

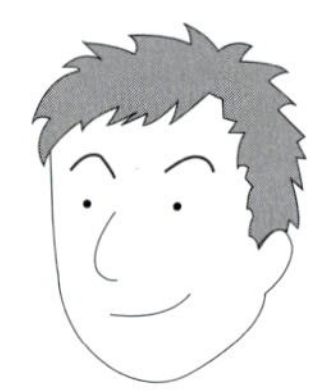

Certainly. (물론이죠.)

Could you spell your name?
(이름의 철자가 어떻게 되세요?)

W-I-N-S-L-E-T.

first visit : 초진　a health insurance card : 건강보험증　spell : 철자하다　in : …에

Grammar

May I… ?	~해도 괜찮을까요?	Certainly. I'm sorry, but…

May I have your name? — 성함이 어떻게 되시죠?
use your phone? — 전화기 좀 사용해도 될까요?
borrow your umbrella? — 우산 좀 빌려 주시겠어요?
smoke here? — 여기서 담배를 피워도 되나요?
help you? — 도와드릴까요?

'Could I…?' 도 정중하게 허락을 얻을 때 쓰는 표현입니다. 'Can I…?' 는 격의 없이 물어보는 표현입니다.

Could you (please)… ?	~해도 괜찮을까요?	Yes, of course. I'm sorry, but…

Could you tell me your work number? — 직장 전화번호를 알려 주시겠어요?

spell your last name? — 이름의 철자를 알려 주시겠어요?

show me your insurance card? — 건강보험증을 보여 주시겠어요?

wait for a while? — 잠깐 기다려 주시겠어요?

help me? — 저를 좀 도와주시겠어요?

'Would you…?' 도 의뢰나 요구를 할 때 쓰는 표현입니다. 이 표현은 'Can you…?' 보다 공손한 말입니다.

Practice

1. 네모 속의 단어를 골라 빈 칸에 넣어 문장을 완성하세요.

borrow	have	smoke	come	ask	use

① May I (   ) you some questions? Certainly.

② May I (   ) your name? Yes, my name is Kate Green.

③ May I (   ) this phone? Yes, of course.

④ May I (   ) your umbrella? No problem. Here it is.

⑤ May I (   ) ? I'm afraid you cannot.

⑥ May I (   ) in? Yes, please.

I'm afraid : 미안하지만~, ~해서 유감입니다.

2. 네모 속의 단어를 골라 빈 칸에 넣어 문장을 완성하세요.

spell	wait	tell	help	show	open

① Could you (   ) the window? Sure.

② Could you (   ) me the time? 10 : 30.

③ Could you (   ) your last name? It's G-R-E-E-N.

④ Could you (   ) me your insurance card? Yes. Here you are.

⑤ Could you (   ) for a while? I'm sorry, but I'm in a hurry.

⑥ Could you (   ) me? Yes, of course.

3. 빈 칸에 'are', 'do', 'may', 'could' 를 넣어 문장을 완성하세요.

① ( ) you wait for a while, please?

② ( ) you have a Korean health insurance card?

③ ( ) I open the window?

④ ( ) you a new patient? Yes, I am. ☞ patient :환자

⑤ ( ) you spell your last name, please?

⑥ ( ) I turn on the light? ☞ turn on/off : (전등이나 텔레비전)을 켜다. / 끄다.

⑦ ( ) you speak Korean? No, I don't.

4. 빈 칸을 채워 문장을 완성하세요.

① Is this your ( ) visit? Yes, it's my first time here.

② ( ) I have your name? My name is Lucy Smith.

③ Could you ( ) your first name? It's *L-U-C-Y.*

④ Do you ( ) a Korean health insurance card? Yes, I do.

⑤ What is your ( ) ? 4 Hongo 5-chome Bunkyo-ku, Tokyo.

⑥ ( ) is your date of birth? July 15, 1955.

⑦ What do you ( ) ? I'm a nurse.

⑧ ( ) you single or married? I'm single.

⑨ What's your ( ) ? I'm American.

5. 상대에게 영어로 질문을 하고, 아래의 진료신청서를 작성하세요.

성 명		직 업	
전 화		결 혼	기혼 · 미혼
생년월일		보 험	유 · 무
현 주 소			
국 적			

UNIT 4 FOCUS

우리말과 영어는 주소, 전화번호, 날짜를 말하는 방법이 서로 다릅니다. 이를 연습해 보세요.

<우리말>

주소	123-456 서울특별시 강남구 삼성동 123번지 정수진
전화번호	00-123-4560
생년월일	1985년 3월 3일

<영어>

ADDRESS	Ms. Soo-Jin Chung 123, Samsung-dong, Gangnam-gu Seoul, 123-456, Republic of Korea
PHONE	00-123-4560 (double oh, one two three, four five six oh)
THE DATE OF BIRTH	March 3, 1985 (March third, nineteen eighty-five)

Answer Key

1 ① ask ② have ③ use ④ borrow ⑤ smoke ⑥ come

2 ① open ② tell ③ spell ④ show ⑤ wait ⑥ help

3 ① Could ② Do ③ May / Could ④ Are ⑤ Could ⑥ May / Could ⑦ Do

4 ① first ② May ③ spell ④ have ⑤ address ⑥ What ⑦ do ⑧ Are ⑨ nationality

UNIT 5 I have a toothache.

Vocabulary

cold	감기	*flu*	인플루엔자(독감)	*cough*	기침
chill	한기	*sore throat*	목이 아픔	*fever*	열
headache	두통	*stomachache*	위통, 복통	*earache*	귀가 아픔
toothache	치통	*backache*	등의 통증, 요통	*sick*	구토

Key sentences

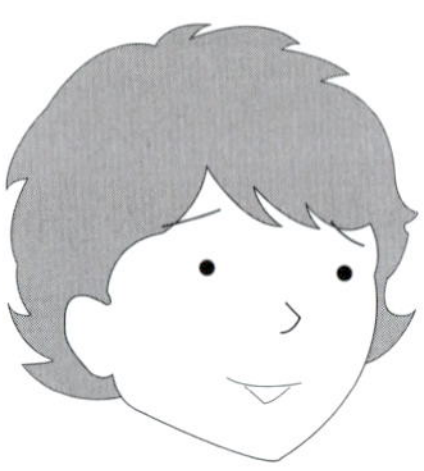

What's the matter?
(무슨 일인가요?)

I have a toothache.
(이가 아픕니다.)

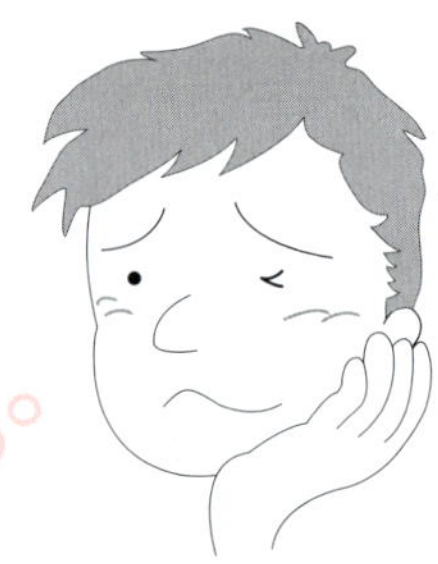

1. 문장 가운데 붉은 색의 단어를 다른 말로 바꾸어 다양한 증상을 표현해 보세요.

I have a cold.	I have a headache.	I have the flu.
a cough.	a stomachache.	I feel sick.
a sore throat.	an earache.	
a chill.	a toothache.	
a fever.	a backache.	

2. ①~⑥의 증상을 영어로 써 보세요.

①
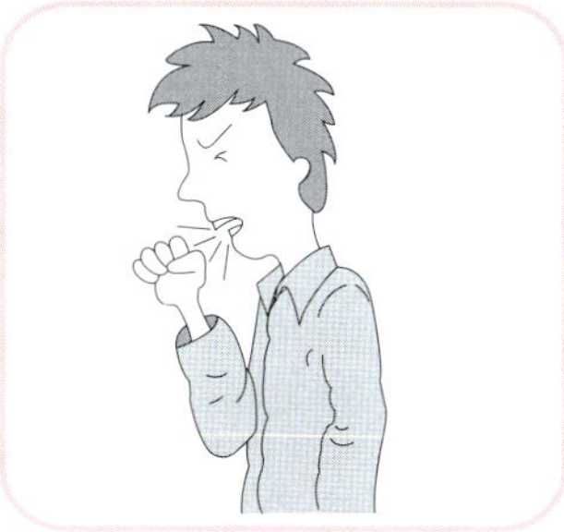
②
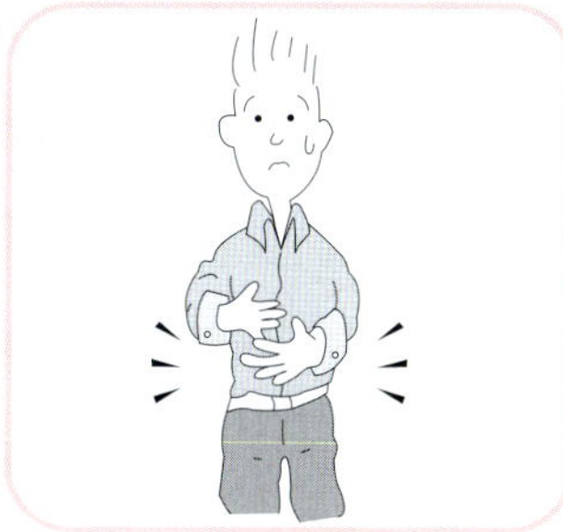
③
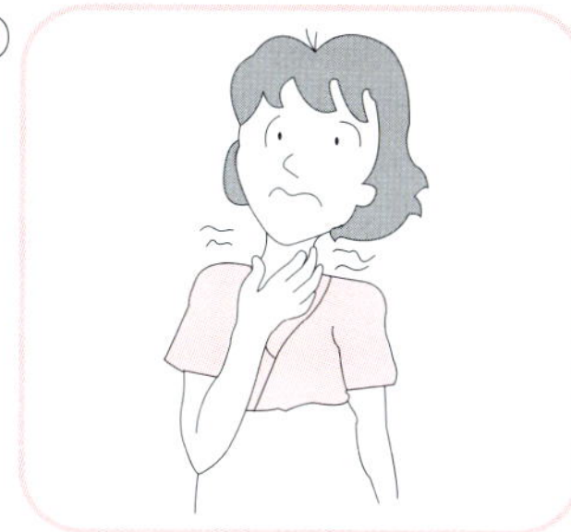

④
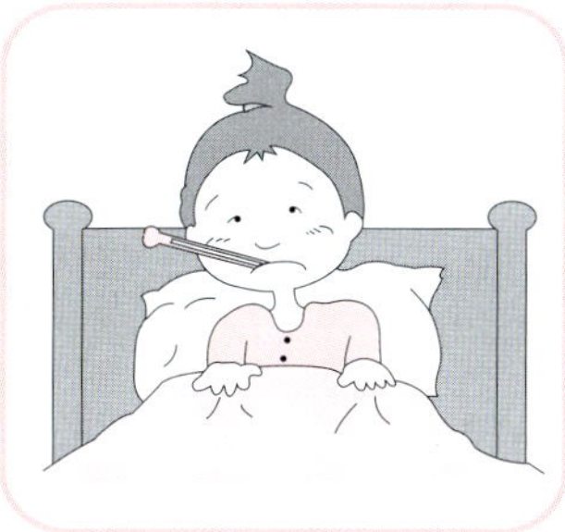
⑤
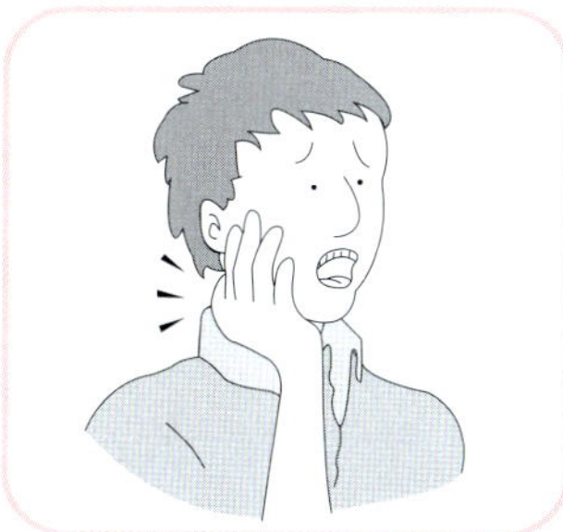
⑥
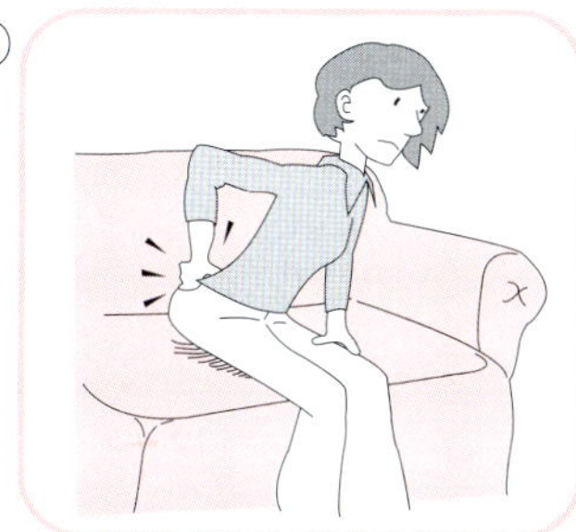

①   ②

③   ④

⑤   ⑥

3. 당신은 감기를 어떻게 치료합니까? 상대에게 영어로 질문해 보세요.

* How do you treat a cold?

① Do you have anything hot?

② Do you eat nutritious food?

③ Do you take a bath?

④ Do you exercise and perspire?

⑤ Do you see a doctor?

⑥ Do you take medicine?

⑦ Do you go to sleep and rest?

	Yes	No
①		
②		
③		
④		
⑤		
⑥		
⑦		

☞ nutritious : 영양가 있는   perspire : 땀을 흘리다   rest : 쉬다   medicine : 약

* 감기는 어떻게 치료합니까? ① 따뜻한 물을 마십니까? ② 영양식을 먹습니까?
③ 목욕을 합니까? ④ 운동을 해서 땀을 흘립니까? ⑤ 의사에게 진료를 받습니까?
⑥ 약을 먹습니까? ⑦ 잠을 자면서 쉬나요?

4. 역할을 나누어 그림의 내용을 보면서 밑줄 친 부분을 표현해 보세요.

A : How are you? (어떠세요?)

B : Not very well. (좋지 않습니다.)

A : What's the matter? (무슨 일인가요?)

B : I have a cold and a fever. (감기에 걸려 열이 납니다.)

A : I recommend you go home and sleep well. (집에 가서서 푹 주무세요.)

☞ What's the matter? : 무슨 일이세요? I recommend : <…하도록> 권하다

①
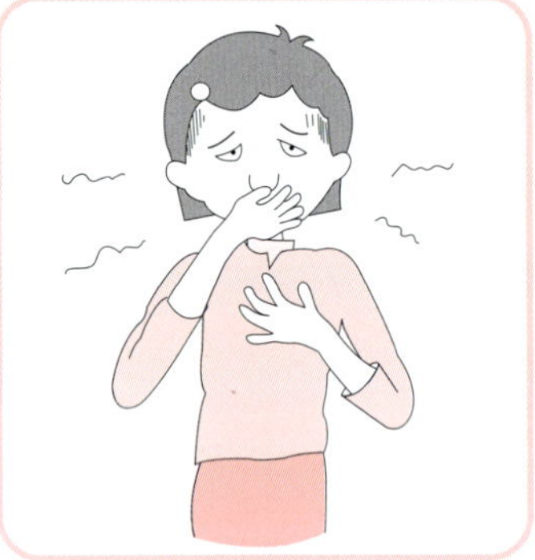

②
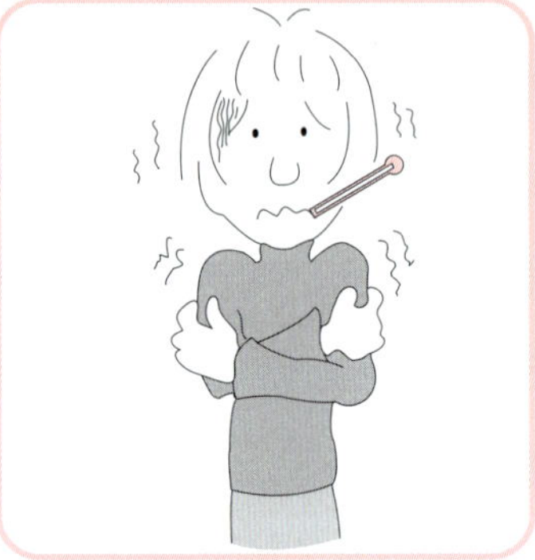

③
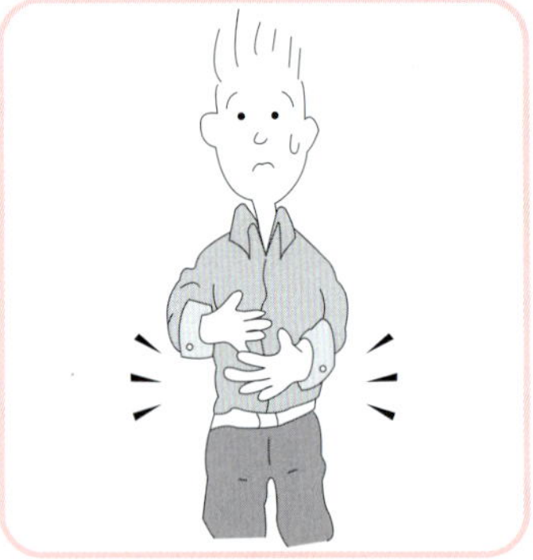

④
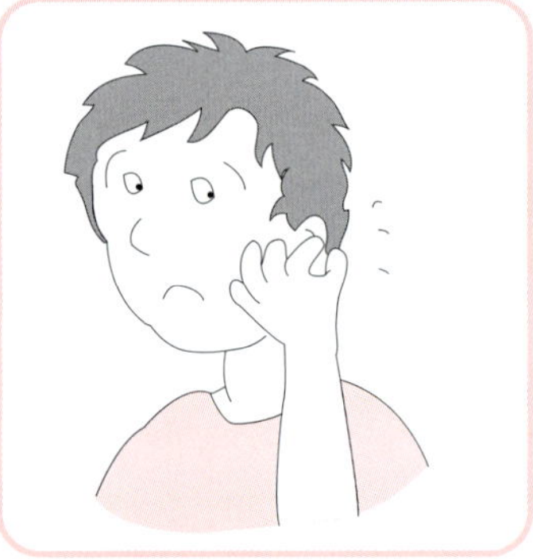

Practice

5. 빈 칸을 채워 문장을 완성하세요.

① I (　　　　　) a headache.

② (　　　　　) you have a cough?

③ She (　　　　　) sick.

④ (　　　　　) she feel sick?

⑤ My son (　　　　　) a toothache.

⑥ (　　　　　) he have a stomachache?

⑦ I have (　　　　　) flu.

⑧ I have (　　　　　) earache.

⑨ (　　　　　) are you? Fine, thank you. And you?

6. 네모 속의 단어를 빈 칸에 넣어 문장을 완성하세요.

sick	matter	toothache	fever	chill

① What's the (　　　　　) ?	I think I have a cold.
② Do you have a (　　　　　) ?	Yes, my temperature is 38°C.
③ Do you have a (　　　　　) ?	Yes, I feel cold.
④ I don't want to eat. I feel (　　　　　).	
⑤ I have a (　　　　　).	Go and see a dentist.

☞ temperature : 체온, 열

Answer Key

2
① I have a cough. ② I have a stomachache. ③ I have a sore throat.
④ I have a fever. ⑤ I have a toothache. ⑥ I have a backache.

4
① B : I feel sick. ② B : I have a chill and a fever.
③ B : I have a stomachache. ④ B : I have an earache.

5
① have ② Do ③ feels ④ Does ⑤ has
⑥ Does ⑦ the ⑧ an ⑨ How

6
① matter ② fever ③ chill ④ sick ⑤ toothache

UNIT 5 FOCUS

「머리가 아프다」 라는 말을 영어로는 "I have a headache." 라고 표현합니다. 영어의 "have" 는 눈에 보이는 것과 보이지 않는 것에 함께 사용할 수 있습니다. 다음의 예처럼 외모를 나타낼 때에도 "have" 를 사용합니다.

I have long hair.

You have blue eyes.

She has beautiful nails.

The elephant has a long nose.

The rabbit has long ears.

영어에는 사람을 처음 만났을 때 상대의 외모를 표현하고 칭찬하는 습관이 있습니다.
역할을 나눠 서로의 외모를 표현하고 칭찬해 봅시다.

You have (a) good ____________________________.

You have (a) beautiful ____________________________.

You have (a) wonderful ____________________________.

이밖에도 have를 사용하여 다음과 같이 표현할 수 있습니다.

I have no idea.	(모르겠습니다.)
I have a dog.	(개를 키우고 있습니다.)
I have breakfast at the cafe.	(카페에서 아침식사를 합니다.)
Have a good time.	(즐거운 시간 가지시길 바랍니다.)
Have a nice trip.	(즐겁게 여행하시길 바랍니다.)

Exercise

다음의 증상이나 용무가 있을 때 어디를 가야 할까요?
(　　) 속에 ①-⑦과 A-G의 뜻을 우리말로 써 보세요. 그리고 짝을 지어 선으로 연결하세요.

① toothache
(　　　　　　　　　　　　　　　　)

② stomachache
(　　　　　　　　　　　　　　　　)

③ sty
(　　　　　　　　　　　　　　　　)

④ rash
(　　　　　　　　　　　　　　　　)

⑤ X-ray
(　　　　　　　　　　　　　　　　)

⑥ payment
(　　　　　　　　　　　　　　　　)

⑦ get your medicine
(　　　　　　　　　　　　　　　　)

A. accounts section
(　　　　　　　　　　　　　　　　)

B. eye clinic
(　　　　　　　　　　　　　　　　)

C. pharmacy
(　　　　　　　　　　　　　　　　)

D. dermatology
(　　　　　　　　　　　　　　　　)

E. radiology
(　　　　　　　　　　　　　　　　)

F. dentistry
(　　　　　　　　　　　　　　　　)

G. internal medicine
(　　　　　　　　　　　　　　　　)

Answer Key

① 치통-F 치과

② 복통-G 내과

③ 다래끼-B 안과

④ 발진-D 피부과

⑤ X선-E 방사선과

⑥ 계산-A 회계

⑦ 약-C 약국

UNIT 6 I'd like to make an appointment for Friday.

Key sentences

I'd like to make an appointment for next Friday morning. (다음 주 금요일 아침에 예약을 했으면 합니다.)

What time would you like to come? (몇 시에 오시기 좋으세요?)

9:00. (9시.)

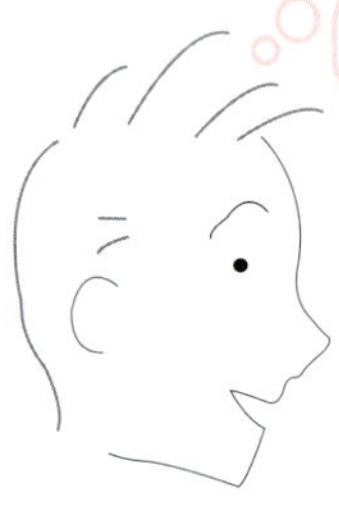

I'm afraid the doctor is busy then. (어쩌지요, 그 시간에는 선생님께서 바쁘신데요.)

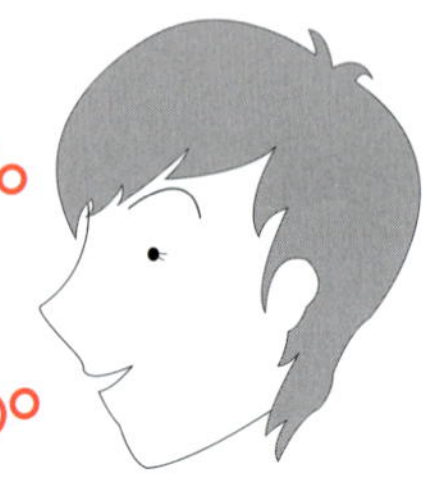

How about 10:30? (10시 30분은 어떠세요?)

Fine. (좋습니다.)

The next appointment is July 15 at 10:30. (다음 예약은 7월 15일, 10시 30분입니다.)

☞ I'd = I would
make an appointment : 예약하다 for : (특정 일시나 기회)…에 busy : 바쁘다

Grammar & Speaking

I would like to …. (가능하다면) …하고 싶은데

I want to see the doctor.	의사에게 진료를 받고 싶어요.
I would like to see the doctor.	의사선생님께 진료를 받을 수 있겠습니까?

✎ "I would like to do" 는 "I want to do"보다 더 정중한 표현입니다.

Would you like to do…? …는 어떻습니까?

Would you like to leave a message?	전할 말씀 있으신가요?
Would you like to go for a drink?	술 한 잔 하러 가시겠습니까?
Would you like to wait a minute?	잠시만 기다려 주시겠습니까?

✎ "Would you like to do?" 는 상대방의 의향을 묻거나(…하고 싶은데), 권유나 제안을 하거나(…하지 않겠습니까?), 정중한 의뢰(…해 주실 수 있을까요?) 등을 표현할 때 사용하는 말입니다.

◆ "do" 부분(동사의 원형)을 바꾸어 연습해 보세요.

I'd like to make an appointment with the doctor.	진료예약을 하고 싶습니다.
ask you some questions.	질문이 있습니다.
cancel my appointment.	예약을 취소하고 싶습니다.
leave here at 11:00.	11시에는 이곳을 떠날 수 있었으면 합니다.

Would you like to come to my house tomorrow?	내일 저의 집에 오실 수 있으시겠어요?
have dinner tonight?	오늘밤에 저녁식사 괜찮으세요?
What would you like to do tonight?	오늘밤 무엇을 하고 싶으신가요?
What time would you like to have dinner?	몇 시에 저녁식사를 하시면 좋으시겠어요?

How about…? …(하면) 어떨까요?

"How about…?" 은 제안이나 권유를 표현합니다.

How about Monday at eleven?	월요일 11시 어떻습니까?
a cup of tea?	차 한 잔 하시겠어요?
going to the movie?	영화 보러 갈까요?
taking a break?	잠깐 쉴까요?

◆ 요일, 월, 날짜, 시간을 표현하는 방법

〈Days of the week〉 요일

Sunday	Monday	Tuesday	Wednesday	Thursday	Friday	Saturday
일요일	월요일	화요일	수요일	목요일	금요일	토요일

〈Months〉 월

January	(1월)	February	(2월)	March	(3월)	April	(4월)
May	(5월)	June	(6월)	July	(7월)	August	(8월)
September	(9월)	October	(10월)	November	(11월)	December	(12월)

〈Date〉 날짜

쓰는 방법	말하는 방법
January 1 / 1st January	January first / the first of January
February 2 / 2nd February	February second / the second of February
April 3 / 3rd April	April third / the third of April

May 4 / 4th May	May fourth / the fourth of May
June 5 / 5th June	June fifth / the fifth of June
July 21 / 21st July	July twenty-first / the twenty first of July
August 30 / 30th August	August thirtieth / the thirtieth of August
1842	eighteen forty-two
1903	nineteen-oh-three
2001	two thousand (and) one
January 14, 2005 = 1/14/05	January fourteenth, two thousand (and) five
14th January 2005 = 14/1/05	the fourteenth of January, two thousand (and) five

<Telling the time> 시간을 말하는 방법

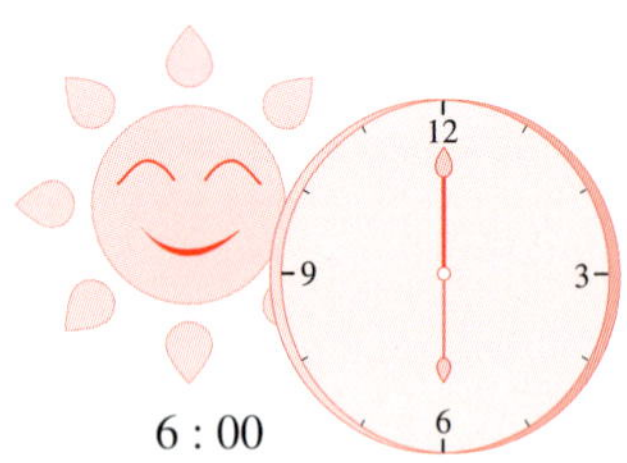

A.M. = a.m.
오전

6 : 00
six o'clock in the morning.
six a.m.

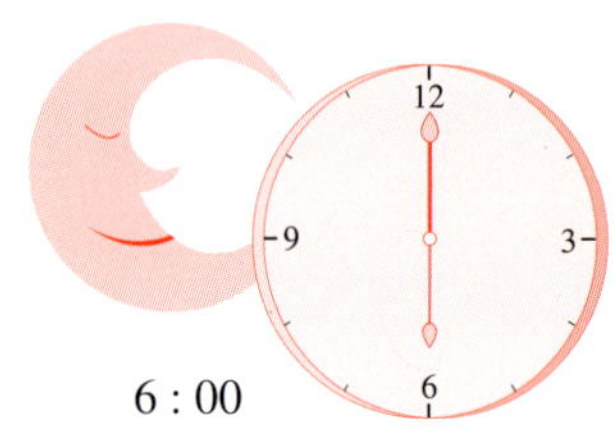

P.M. = p.m.
오후

6 : 00
six o'clock in the evening.
six p.m.

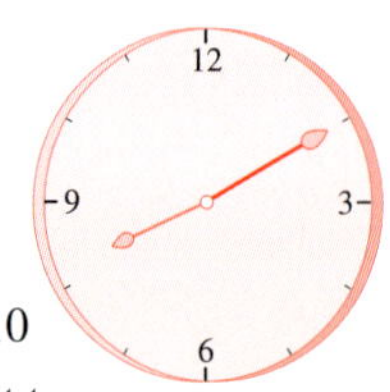

8 : 10
eight ten
ten (minutes) after eight
ten (minutes) past eight

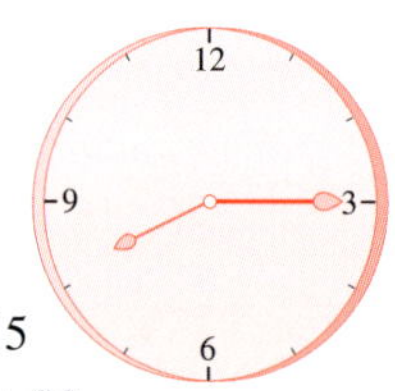

8 : 15
eight fifteen
a quarter after eight
a quarter past eight

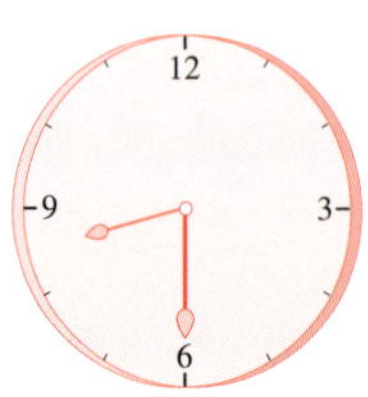

8 : 30
eight thirty
half past eight

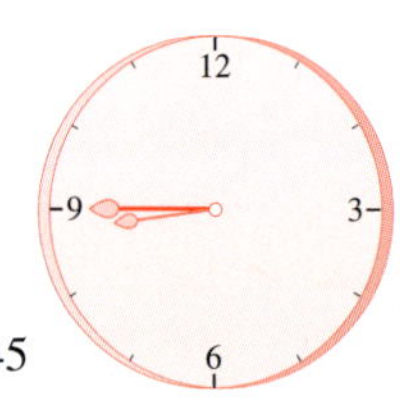

8 : 45
eight forty-five
a quarter to nine
a quarter of nine

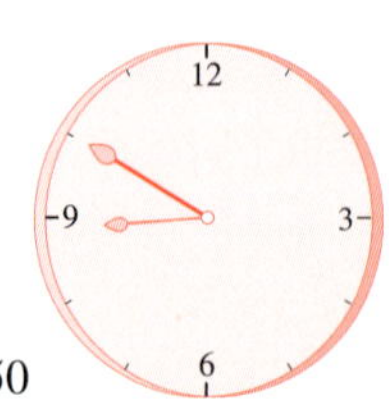

8 : 50
eight fifty
ten (minutes) to nine
ten (minutes) of nine

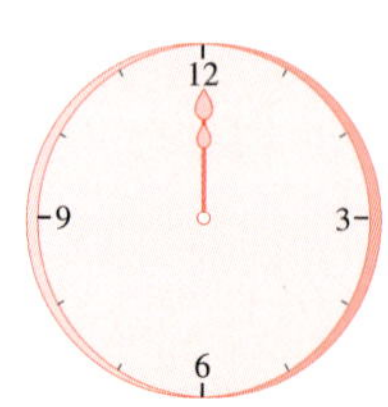

12 : 00
12 a.m. twelve noon
12 p.m. twelve midnight

Practice

1. 빈 칸을 채워 문장을 완성하세요.

① A : I'd like to (　　　　　) an appointment for next Friday morning.

② B : All right. (　　　　　) time would you like to come?

A : 10 : 00 a.m.

③ B : I'm afraid the doctor is (　　　　　) then. How (　　　　　) 10 : 30?

A : Yes. That's fine.

B : Your appointment is Friday, July 13 at 10 : 30.

2. 다음의 시계를 보고 영어로 시간을 표현해 보세요.

① 2 : 50

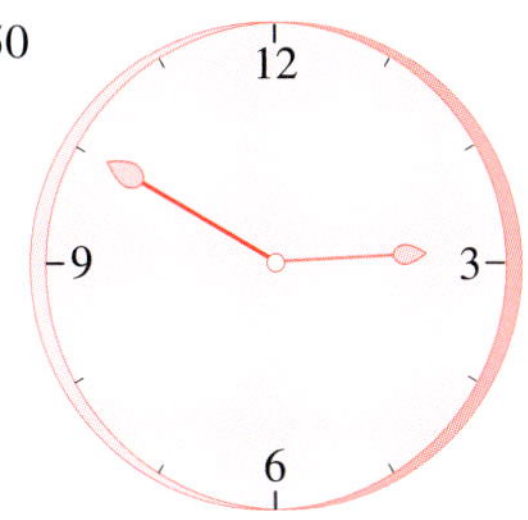

② 3 : 45

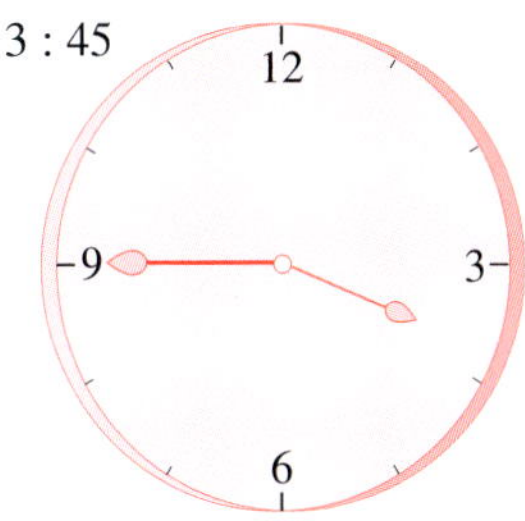

③ 11 : 30

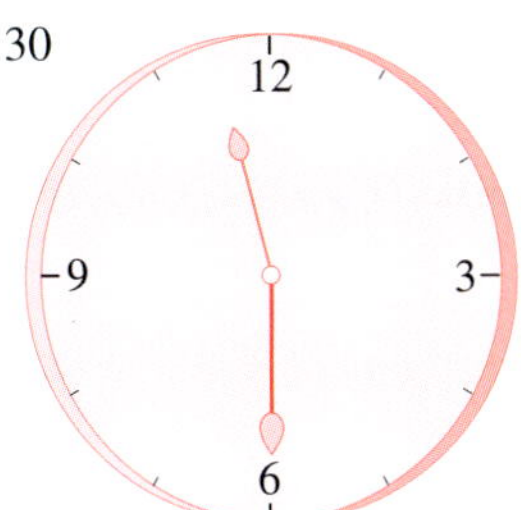

④ 4 : 15

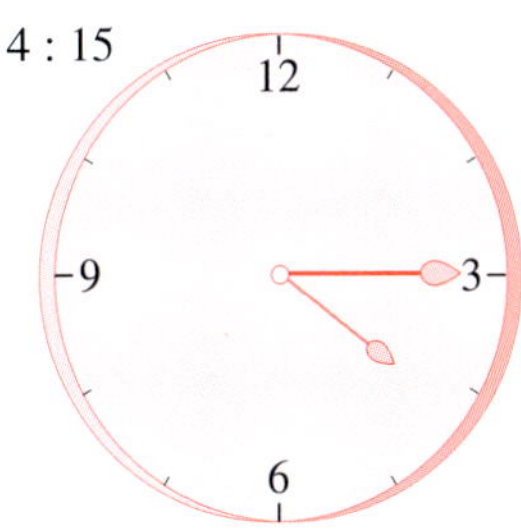

Answer Key

1 ① make　② What　③ busy　④ about

2 ① (It's) two fifty. / (It's) ten (minutes) to three. / (It's) ten (minutes) of three.

② (It's) three forty-five. / (It's) a quarter to four. / (It's) a quarter of four.

③ (It's) eleven thirty. / (It's) half past eleven.

④ (It's) four fifteen. / (It's) a quarter after four. / (It's) a quarter past four.

UNIT 6 FOCUS

전화로 진료예약을 하기도 합니다. 전화통화의 표현을 연습해 보세요.

(1)	This is Kim's Dental Clinic.	(안녕하세요, 김치과입니다.)
(2)	Can I speak to Dr. Kim?	(김 선생님과 통화할 수 있나요?)
(3)	Hold on. Just a moment, please.	(잠시 기다려 주세요.)
(4)	Let me check it out.	(확인해 보겠습니다.)
(5)	The doctor is out. The doctor is not here at the moment.	(선생님은 지금 자리에 안 계십니다.)
(6)	Could you call back later, please?	(조금 후에 다시 전화주시겠습니까?)
(7)	Would you like to leave a message?	(전하실 말씀이 있으신지요?)
(8)	Could you slow down, please?	(천천히 말씀해 주시겠습니까?)
(9)	Could you speak louder, please?	(좀 더 큰 소리로 말씀해 주시겠어요?)
(10)	Thank you very much. Bye.	(감사합니다. 안녕히 계세요.)

Exercise

역할을 나누어 예약하는 연습을 해 보세요.
치과위생사의 역할을 맡은 사람은 A의 일정을 보면서 날짜와 시간을 조정하여 예약을 받습니다.
환자의 역할은 맡은 사람은 B의 일정을 보면서 예약을 합니다.

A. 병원의 일정

	9	10	11	3	4	5
MON	김 선생님		이 선생님			정 선생님
TUE				박 선생님		
WED	전 선생님	장 선생님			조 선생님	
THU				휴진		
FRI	최 선생님			오 선생님		

B. 환자의 일정

	9	10	11	3	4	5
MON	출장 (business trip for Seoul)					
TUE						
WED					고객과 만남 (meeting with clients)	
THU		회의 (meeting in the office)				
FRI		점심식사 약속 (lunch with managers)				

UNIT 7 This tooth is decayed.

Vocabulary

1. *tooth decay (dental caries)*	충치, 치아우식증
2. *a decayed tooth*	충치(썩은 치아)
3. *a cavity*	충치(구멍)
4. *a false tooth (false teeth = dentures)*	의치
5. *a permanent tooth*	영구치
6. *a milk tooth / a baby tooth* *(= a deciduous tooth)*	유치

1. 아래 단어의 뜻을 사전에서 찾아보세요.

① decay

② false

③ cavity

④ permanent

Key sentences

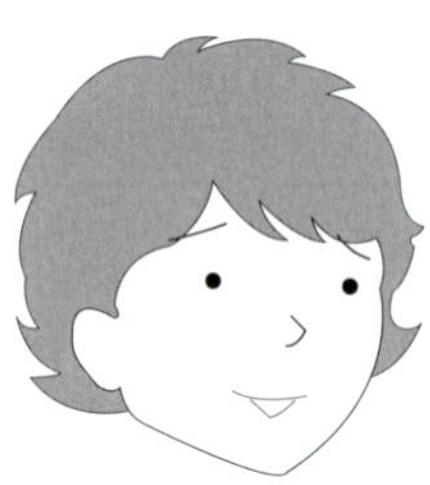

This tooth is decayed.
(이 치아가 썩었군요.)

There are two cavities.
(충치가 두 개 있습니다.)

2. 네모 속의 단어를 골라 문장을 완성하세요.

decayed	baby	cavity	permanent	dentures

① There is a hole in the tooth. I think it's a (   ) .

② This tooth is (   ) .

③ Your (   ) need repairing.

④ Young children have (   ) teeth.

⑤ Milk teeth are replaced by (   ) teeth.

☞ ① 치아에 구멍이 났습니다. 충치 같습니다. ② 이 치아가 썩었군요. ③ 당신의 의치는 수리가 필요합니다.
④ 어린아이들은 유치가 있습니다. ⑤ 유치는 영구치로 바뀝니다.

Vocabulary 2

1.	*upper teeth*	윗니
2.	*lower teeth*	아랫니
3.	*front teeth* (*incisors*)	전치(절치), 앞니
4.	*canine* (*cuspid*)	견치, 송곳니
5.	*back teeth* (*molars and premolars*)	구치(소구치와 대구치), 어금니
6.	*wisdom tooth* (*third molar*)	지치(제3대구치), 사랑니
7.	*gum* (*gingiva*) / *gums* (*gingivae*)	치은, 잇몸
8.	*enamel*	법랑질
9.	*pulp*	치수
10.	*dentine*	상아질
11.	*tongue*	혀

3. 네모 속의 단어를 골라 ( )에 각각의 명칭을 써 보세요.

upper teeth
lower teeth
canine
front teeth
back teeth
tongue

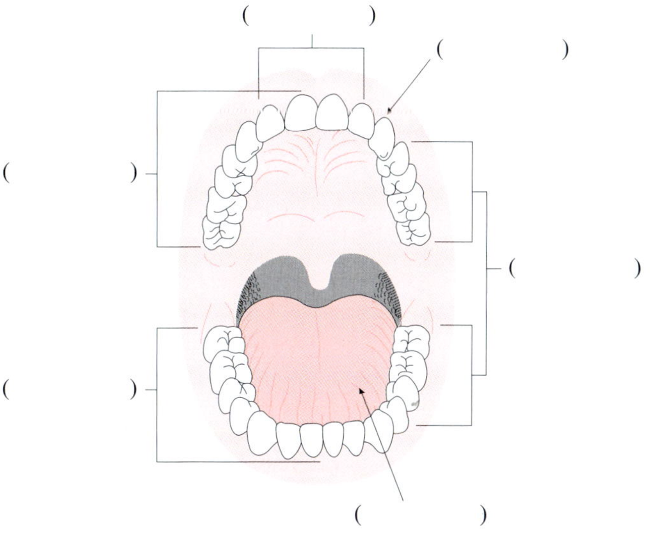

enamel
dentine
pulp
gum

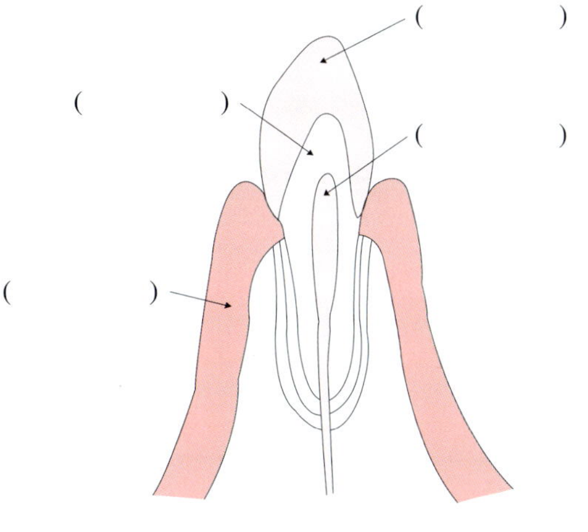

4. 네모 속의 단어를 사용해 치아에 관한 문장을 완성하세요.

enamel	back	pulp	lower	wisdom	upper	canine	front

① Incisors are (   ) teeth.

② Molars and premolars are (   ) teeth.

③ There are four (   ) teeth in the mouth.

④ A (   ) is between the front teeth and the back teeth.

⑤ There is (   ) on dentine.

⑥ You have lips, an (   ) lip and a (   ) lip.

⑦ There is (   ) in the center of a tooth.

5. 전문용어를 환자가 이해하기 쉬운 영어로 고쳐 빈 칸에 써 보세요.

환자가 이해하기 쉬운 용어		전문용어
치아우식증(충치)		dental caries
치은		gingiva
전치		incisor
구치		molar/premolar
유치		deciduous tooth
지치		third molar
견치		cuspid

6. 네모 속의 단어를 골라 빈 칸을 채워 문장을 완성하세요.

gums	back	front	wisdom

① An upper (   ) tooth was chipped while eating.

② Your (   ) are swollen.

③ I think I have to extract your (   ) tooth.

④ Do you brush your (   ) teeth carefully?

☞ 1) 식사 중에 윗니가 빠졌어요.   2) 잇몸이 부었군요.
3) 사랑니를 빼야겠군요.   4) 어금니는 꼼꼼하게 닦나요?

7. (   )에 알맞은 동사를 네모에서 골라 문장을 완성하세요.

bleed	brush	extract	have

① I (   ) a toothache.

② I'm going to (   ) the nerve of the tooth.

③ Do your gums (   ) ?

④ Do you (   ) your teeth properly?

☞ be going to… : …할 생각이다   nerve : 신경   bleed : 피가 난다   properly : 적절히, 바르게

Answer Key

2 ① cavity ② decayed ③ dentures ④ baby/milk/deciduous
⑤ permanent

4 ① front ② back ③ wisdom ④ canine ⑤ enamel
⑥ upper, lower ⑦ pulp

5 썩은 이(충치) : tooth decay 잇몸 : gum 앞니 : front tooth
어금니 : back tooth 젖니 : baby tooth 또는 milk tooth
사랑니 : wisdom tooth 송곳니 : canine

6 ① front ② gums ③ wisdom ④ back

7 ① have ② extract ③ bleed ④ brush

FOCUS

영어는 「하나(단수)」와 「둘 이상(복수)」을 구별하여 표현합니다. 사물이 둘 이상일 때에는 단어의 형태가 바뀝니다. 어떻게 바뀌는지 확인하세요.

	단 수	복 수
① 자음 + y → -ies	candy dictionary	
② -o,-s, -z, -x, ch, sh → -es	tomato box	
③ ①, ②, ④ 이외 → -s	book ball	
④ 발음, 형태가 모두 바뀜	child knife	

영어에서는 사물을 「셀 수 있는 것」과 「셀 수 없는 것」으로 구별하여 표현합니다. 영어사전을 찾을 때 'c'라는 표시는 countable, 즉 「셀 수 있음」을 나타냅니다. 이에 비해 'u' 라는 표시는 uncountable, 즉 「셀 수 없음」을 나타냅니다.

다음에 예로 든 사물은 셀 수 있을까요? 사전을 찾아 셀 수 있는 것은 c, 셀 수 없는 것은 u라고 ( )에 쓰세요.

1. money ( )	6. sugar ( )
2. coin ( )	7. water ( )
3. paper ( )	8. rice ( )
4. file ( )	9. bread ( )
5. egg ( )	10. cookie ( )

Answer Key

① candies, dictionaries ② tomatoes, boxes ③ books, balls ④ children, knives

1. u 2. c 3. u 4. c 5. c 6. u 7. u 8. u 9. u 10.c

Exercise

「~(사물)이 ~(장소)에 있습니다.」라는 표현에는 There is…/There are…라고 정해진 형태가 있습니다. 사물이 「하나 」이거나 그 수를 「셀 수 없을」 때에는 There is…를 사용합니다. 사물이 「둘 이상」 일 때에는 There are…를 사용합니다.

There	BE	사물	장소
There	is	a book	on the desk.
There	is	a book	under the table.
There	is	wine	in the bottle.
There	is	salt	in the pot.
There	are	ten books	on the shelf.
There	are	many books	in the library.

(　　)안에 is, are를 넣어 보세요. 「사물」에 주목하여 생각해 보세요.

1. There (　　　　) water in the bottle.
2. There (　　　　) a lot of candies in the bag.
3. There (　　　　) some dogs in the garden.
4. There (　　　　) many students in the classroom.
5. There (　　　　) an apple on the plate.
6. There (　　　　) elephants in the zoo.
7. There (　　　　) paper on the tray.
8. There (　　　　) glasses on the table.
9. There (　　　　) a lot of snow in my yard.
10. There (　　　　) some sugar in the drawer.

이러한 문장은 특정한 사물(my books, your wine, the dictionary 등)에는 사용할 수 없습니다.

× There is Disney land in Japan.
× There are my books in my bag.
× There is your wine in the refrigerator.
× There is the files of the patient on the desk.

Answer Key

1. is　2. are　3. are　4. are　5. is　6. are　7. is　8. are　9. is　10. is

UNIT 8 Parts of the Body

Vocabulary

head	머리	*forehead*	이마	*eye*	눈	*eyebrow*	눈썹
ear	귀	*nose*	코	*mouth*	입	*lip*	입술
cheek	뺨	*jaw*	턱	*chin*	턱 끝	*neck*	목
shoulder	어깨	*arm*	팔	*back*	등	*chest*	가슴
waist	허리	*leg*	다리	*foot*	발	*hip*	엉덩이, 고관절부

☞ hip : 허리 아래에 좌우로 튀어나온 부분

1. ( )에 신체 부위를 영어로 써 보세요.

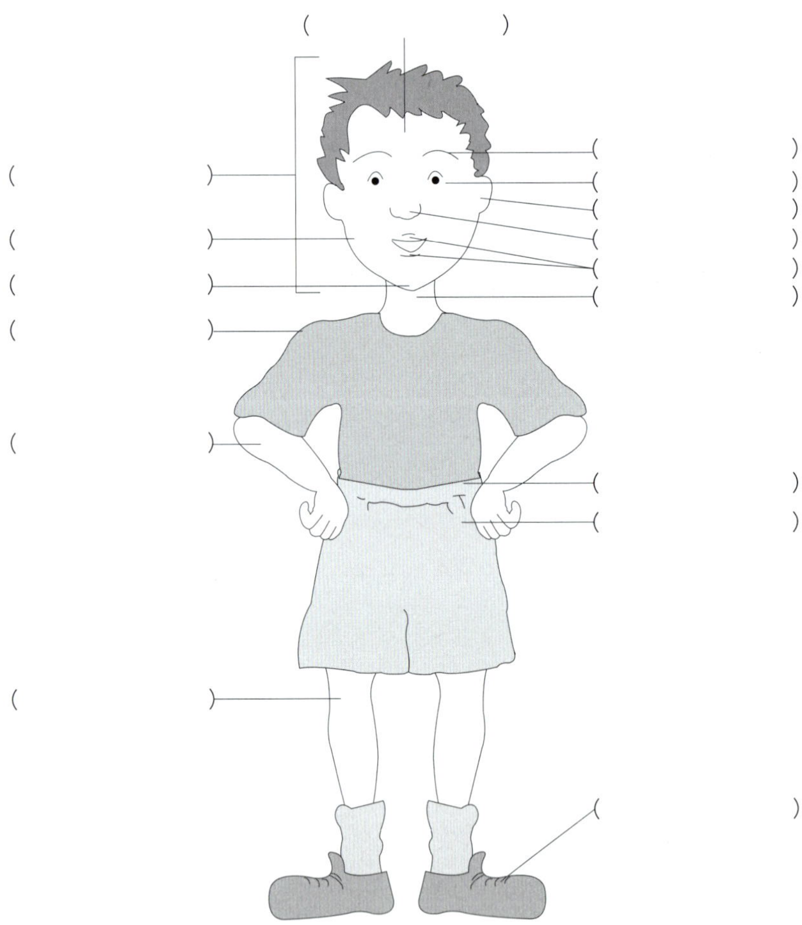

finger	손가락	*thumb*	엄지	*forefinger*	검지
middle finger	중지	*ring finger*	약지	*little finger*	새끼손가락
palm	손바닥	*finger nail*	손톱		

fingers

(   )
(   )
(   )
(   )

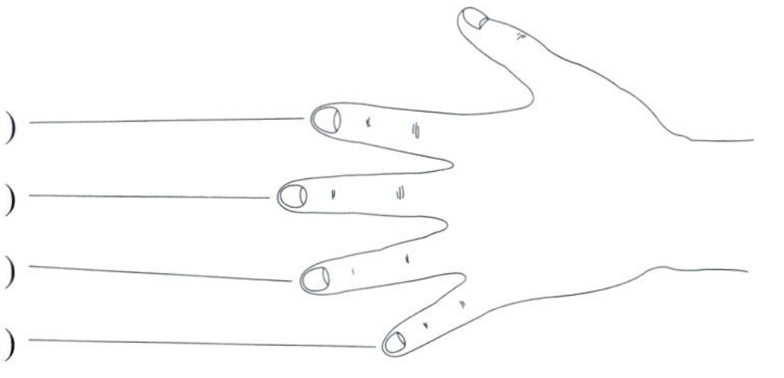

2. 몸동작을 기억하세요.

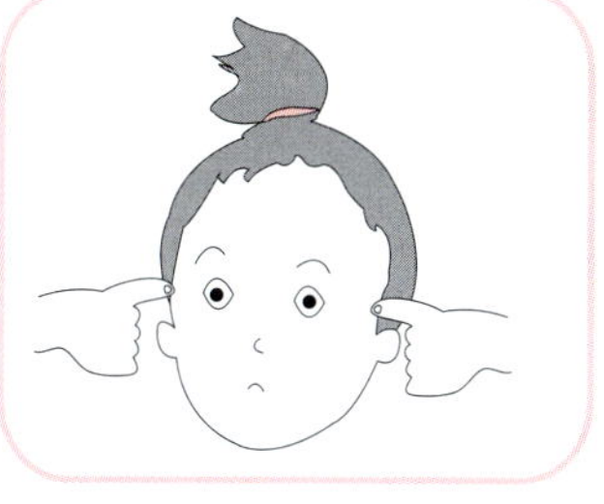

Point to your eyes.

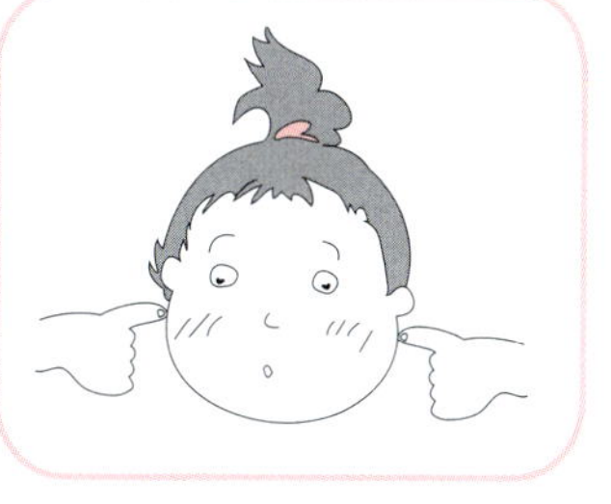

Point to your cheeks.

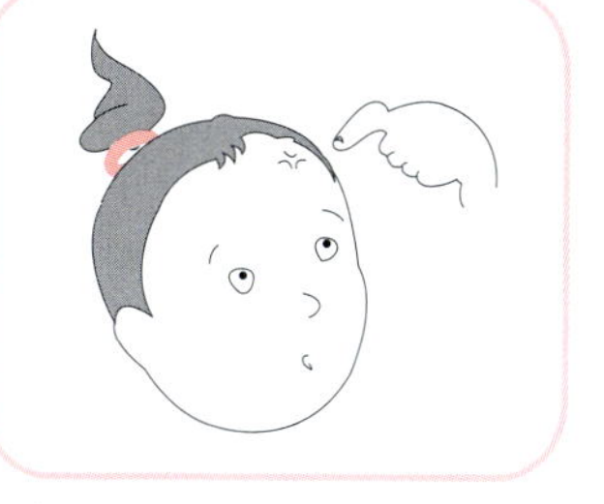

Point to your forehead.

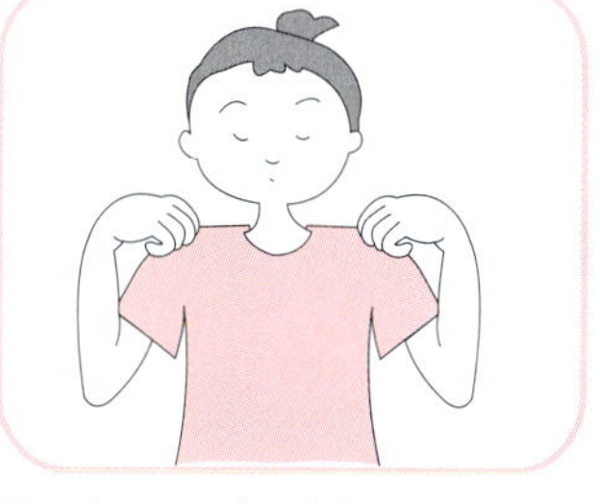

Touch your shoulders.

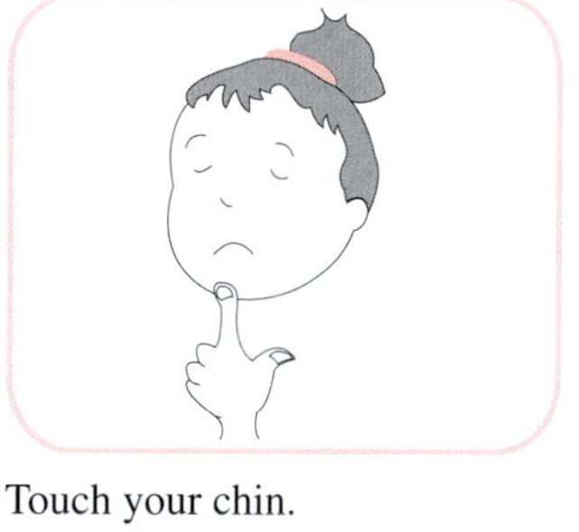

Touch your chin.

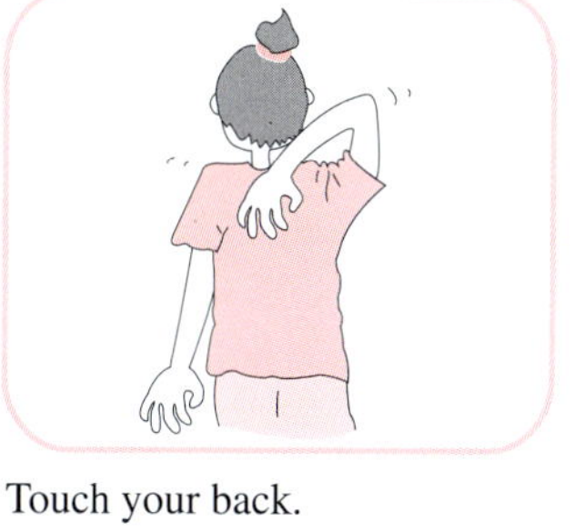

Touch your back.

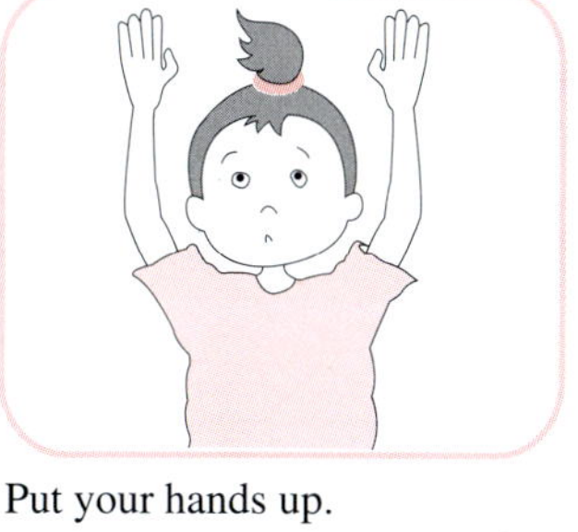

Put your hands up.

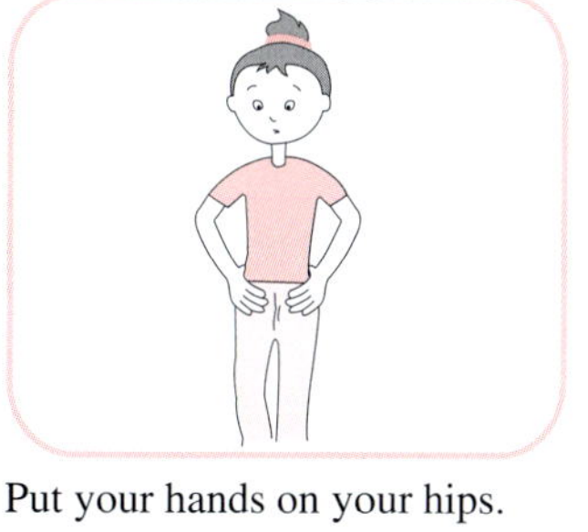

Put your hands on your hips.

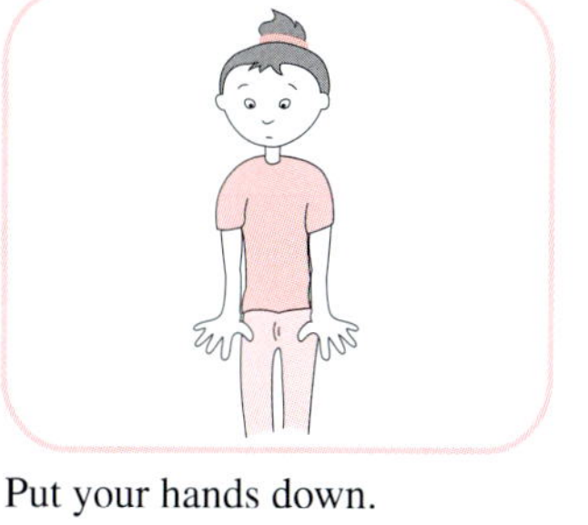

Put your hands down.

☞ point to… : (…)을 가리키다   touch : (…을) 만지다   put : (…을) 두다

3. 선생님이 다음과 같이 영어로 지시를 합니다. 지시에 따라 움직이세요.

1) Stand up.

2) Point to your eyes. / cheeks / chin / forehead, etc.

3) Touch your head. / ears / eyebrows / chest, etc.

4) Put your hands up. / down / on your hips / on your shoulders, etc.

5) Put your right hand on your head. / on your waist, etc.

6) Sit down.

◆ 키와 몸무게를 묻는 방법

[height] 키

A : How tall are you? / What is your height? (키는 얼마나 되나요?)

B : I'm 165 centimeters tall.

[weight] 몸무게

A : How much do you weigh? / What is your weight? (몸무게는 얼마나 되나요?)

B : I weigh 55 kilograms.

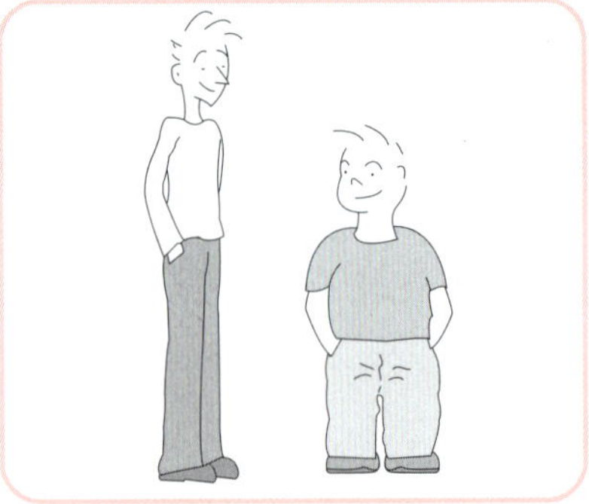

tall ⇔ short

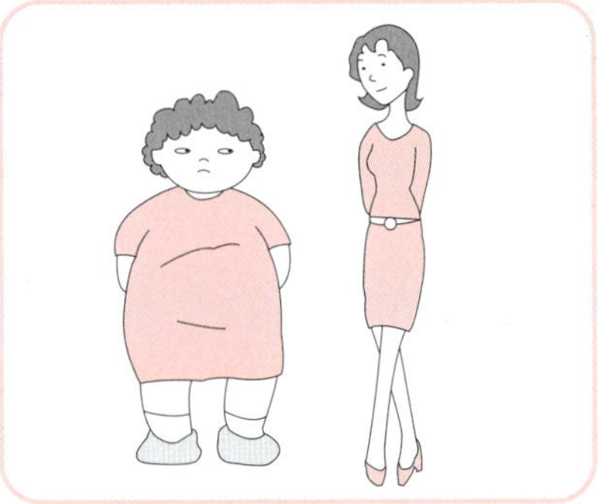

overweight ⇔ slim

Practice

4. 빈 칸을 채우세요.

① He isn't tall. He's (   ).

② She isn't slim. She's (   ).

③ How (   ) (   ) she?   She's 159 cm tall.

④ How (   ) (   ) he weigh?   He weighs 65 kg.

5. 우리 몸에 두개가 있는 것은 무엇일까요? 하나뿐인 것에는 X를, 둘이 있는 것에는 그 복수형을 ( )에 써 보세요.

① head	( )	⑥ neck	( )
② nose	( )	⑦ arm	( )
③ eye	( )	⑧ hand	( )
④ lip	( )	⑨ leg	( )
⑤ mouth	( )	⑩ finger	( )

☞ 영어에서는 「하나」, 「둘 이상」을 분명하게 표시합니다.

Answer Key

4 ① short ② overweight ③ tall, is ④ much, does

5 ① × ② × ③ eyes ④ lips ⑤ × ⑥ × ⑦ arms ⑧ hands ⑨ legs ⑩ fingers

UNIT 8 FOCUS

「얼마나 [ ] 입니까?」 라는 질문과 이를 대답하는 방법을 확인해 보세요.

A : How [ ] are you?

B : I'm (숫자) (단위) [ ].

(예1) A : How old are you?

B : I'm (seventeen) (years) old.

(seventeen) = 숫자, (years) = 단위

(예2) A : How tall are you?

B : I'm (one hundred sixty five) (centimeters) tall.

(one hundred sixty five) = 숫자, (centimeters) = 단위

숫자가 복수(둘 이상)일 때에는 그의 단위도 함께 복수가 됩니다.

× I'm twenty year old.

○ I'm twenty years old.

× I'm one hundred and sixty five centimeter tall.

○ I'm one hundred and sixty five centimeters tall.

주의! 영어에서는 meter, centimeter의 미터법을 사용하지 않고 mile(miles), foot(feet), inch(inches)로 높이와 길이를 나타냅니다.

1 mile = 1603 meters
1 foot = 30.43 centimeters
1 inch = 2.54 centimeters

(예) The river is one thousand miles long.
I'm six feet tall.
The rope is nine inches long.

Exercise

「얼마나 …?」라는 질문과 이를 대답하는 방법을 연습해 보세요.

1. 네모 속의 단어를 골라 (1)~(4)의 빈 칸에 넣어 문장을 완성하세요.

long	high	deep

How (1) is Mt. Halla? It is 1,950 meters (1).

How (2) is Tokyo Tower? It is 333 meters (2).

How (3) is the Bay Bridge? It is 860 meters (3).

How (4) is the Han River? It is 10 meters (4).

2. 여러분 주위에 있는 사물에 대해 대답해 보세요.

(1) How long is your pen?

(2) How tall is your teacher?

(3) How wide is the blackboard in your classroom?

3. 친구와 역할을 나누어 「얼마나…?」를 넣어 질문해 보세요.

(1) ______________________________

(2) ______________________________

(3) ______________________________

Answer Key

1 (1) high (2) high (3) long (4) deep

UNIT 9 Where does it hurt?

Vocabulary

pain 통증

severe pain	심한 통증
sharp pain	날카로운 통증(예통)
throbbing pain	욱신거리는 통증
dull pain	둔한 통증(둔통)

ache 통증

toothache	치통
headache	두통
stomachache	위통, 복통
backache	등의 통증, 요통
earache	귀의 통증

1. 좌우의 문장이 같은 뜻이 되도록 빈 칸에 알맞은 단어를 쓰세요.

I have a toothache. = I have a pain in my (tooth).

I have a stomachache. = I have a pain in my ( ).

I have a backache. = I have a pain in my ( ).

I have an earache. = I have a pain in my ( ).

Key sentences

<통증에 대한 질문>

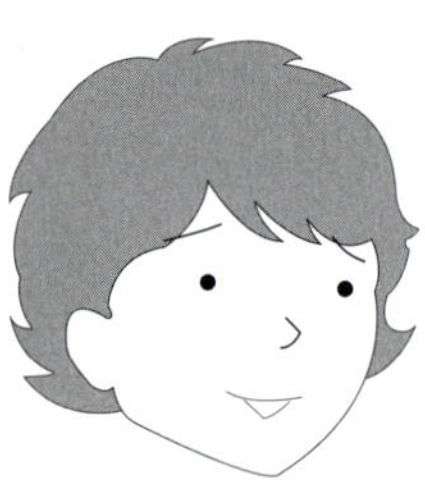

Where does it hurt? (어디가 아픈가요?)
(Where is the pain?)

How long have you had the pain?
(통증이 얼마나 오랫동안 있었나요?)

What kind of pain is it? (어떠한 통증입니까?)

When does it hurt? (언제 아픕니까?)

Is it sensitive to cold water? (차가운 물에 민감하세요?)

Grammar

How long have you~ ?　　~는 얼마나 오랫동안 계속되었나요?

[I have a toothache.]

How long have you had a toothache?
(치통이 얼마나 오랫동안 있었나요?)

For two days.
(이틀 동안이요.)
Since yesterday.
(어제부터요)

[I am sick.]

How long have you been sick?
(아픈지 얼마나 되었나요?)

Practice

2. "How long" (~은 얼마나 오랫동안 계속되었나요?)으로 시작하는 의문문을 만드세요.

① I have pain. ⇒ How long have you had pain?

② I have a headache. ⇒

③ I am smoking. ⇒

④ My gums are swollen. ⇒

⑤ He is waiting. ⇒

⑥ I work at the bank. ⇒

3. 아래 질문의 대답을 오른쪽에서 골라 선으로 연결하세요.

What's the matter?	⇒	· It's a sharp pain.
Where does it hurt?	⇒	· Yes, it is.
What kind of pain is it?	⇒	· For two days.
Is it sensitive to cold water?	⇒	· Here.
How long have you had the pain?	⇒	· I have a toothache.

4. 역할을 나누어 치과위생사 역할을 맡은 사람이 1~5의 질문을 영어로 묻고, 환자의 역할을 맡은 사람이 환자 A가 되어 대답합니다. 그 다음에는 역할을 서로 바꾸어 환자 B가 되어 연습을 하세요.

1. 어떻게 오셨습니까? ____________________

2. 어디가 아프세요? ____________________

3. 어떻게 아프십니까? ____________________

4. 찬 물이 닿으면 시리십니까? ____________________

5. 아픈지 얼마나 되셨습니까? ____________________

〈 patient (환자) A 〉

1. I have a toothache.
2. I have a pain in my back tooth.
3. It's a severe pain.
4. Yes.
5. Since yesterday.

〈 patient B 〉

1. The gum is swollen.
2. The upper gum hurts.
3. I have a dull pain.
4. No, but I feel pain when I eat hard food.
5. For a week.

Answer Key

1

I have a stomachache.	=	I have a pain in my (stomach) .
I have a backache.	=	I have a pain in my (back) .
I have an earache.	=	I have a pain in my (ear) .

2

② How long have you had a headache?

③ How long have you been smoking?

④ How long have your gums been swollen?

⑤ How long has he been waiting?

⑥ How long have you worked at the bank?

3

What's the matter?	— I have a toothache.
Where does it hurt?	— Here.
What kind of pain is it?	— It's a sharp pain.
Is it sensitive to cold water?	— Yes, it is
How long have you had the pain?	— For two days.

현재형과 과거형, 완료형의 차이를 확인합시다.

<형태의 차이>

① 현재형(동사의 현재형)	I	have	a toothache.
② 과거형(동사의 과거형)	I	had	a toothache.
③ 완료형(have+동사의 과거분사)	I	have **had** (과거분사)	a toothache.

(예제) (　)의 동사를 사용하여 빈 칸을 채우세요. 형태는 과거분사입니다.

I have ____________ in Seoul. (live)

I have ____________ English. (study)

<의미의 차이>

① 현재형 · ② 과거형

둥근 점은 사건이 일어난 시기를 말합니다.

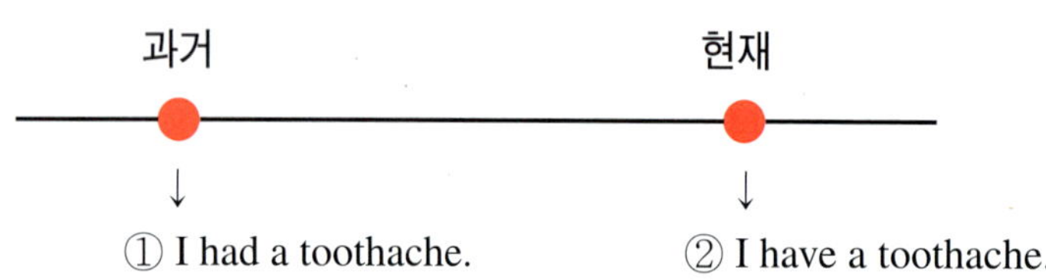

③ 완료형

과거부터 현재까지 계속해서 일어난 사건을 나타냅니다.

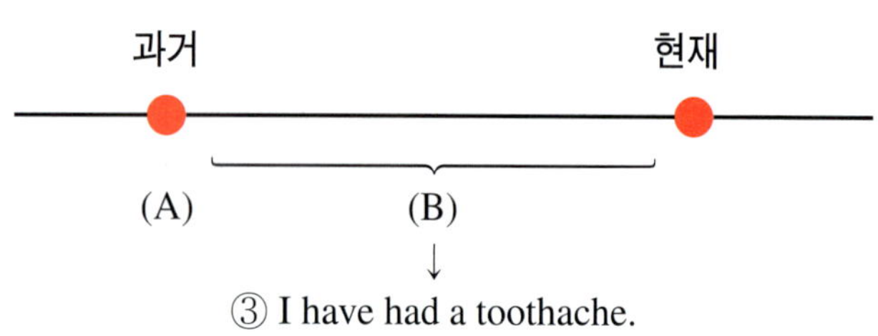

기간을 나타내는 표현에는 두 가지가 있습니다.

· 기간의 출발시점(A)에서 표현합니다. I have had a toothache **since** yesterday.

· 기간의 길이(B)로 표현합니다. I have had a toothache **for** two days.

Answer Key

(예제) lived, studied

Exercise

1. 자신의 경험으로 다음의 질문에 답을 하세요.

(1) Do you like English?

Have you studied English only in your school?

How long have you studied English?

(2) Where were you born?

Where do you live now?

How long have you lived there?

(3) Do you like sports?

What kind of sports do you play?

How long have you played it?

2. 역할을 바꾸어 상대의 취미를 질문해 보세요.

(1) 취미는 무엇입니까? (현재형)

(2) 언제 시작하셨습니까? (과거형)

(3) 얼마나 오랫동안 해오셨습니까? (완료형)

Answer Key

2

(1) What's your hobby?

(2) When did you start it?

(3) How long have you been doing it?

UNIT 10 I'd like to ask you about your medical history.

Vocabulary

medical history	병력	
illness	질병	a serious illness : 중병
allergy	알레르기	
medicine	약	take medicine : 약을 먹다

Key sentences

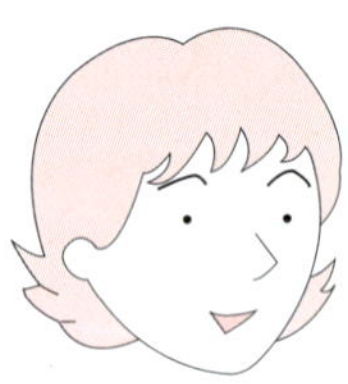

I'd like to ask you about your medical history.
(병력에 대해 여쭤보겠습니다.)

Are you in good health? (건강은 좋으십니까?)

Have you ever had a serious illness?
(심각한 질병을 앓은 적이 있습니까?)

Do you have any allergies? (알레르기가 있습니까?)

Are you taking any medicine? (약을 복용하고 있습니까?)

Grammar

Have you (ever) … ?　「…한 적이 있습니까?」

<have+과거분사>는 현재까지의 경험을 표현하는 현재완료형입니다.

Have you ever **been** to France?	프랑스에 간 적이 있습니까?
read that book?	저 책을 읽은 적이 있습니까?
flown in a plane?	비행기를 타 본 적이 있습니까?
lost your wallet?	지갑을 잃어버린 적이 있습니까?
No, never. (=I have never been to France.)	전혀 없습니다.
Yes, many times. (=I have been to France many times.)	여러 번 있습니다.
Yes, once.	한 번 있습니다.
Yes, twice.	두 번 있습니다.
Yes, a few times.	몇 번 있습니다.

Practice

1. ( ) 속의 단어를 정확한 형태로 만들어 문장을 완성하세요.

① (be) I've never ___been___ to this office.

② (meet) Have you ever ___________ him?

③ (eat) Have you ever ___________ kimchi?

④ (visit) I have never ___________ the dentist for a checkup.

⑤ (see) Have you ever ___________ this cell phone?

⑥ (write) Have you ever ___________ a letter to your parents?

⑦ (lose) My grandfather has never ___________ his teeth.

☞ I've = I have checkup : 검사 cell phone : 휴대전화

2. ( ) 속의 단어를 사용하여 "Have you ever"로 시작하는 의문문을 만들어 보세요.

1. (have an operation)

____ ?

2. (have a dental checkup)

____ ?

3. (be sick during dental treatment)

____ ?

4. (care about your bad breath)

____ ?

5. (be here)

____ ?

☞ have an operation : 수술을 받다 during dental treatment : 치과치료 중
care about : ~을 걱정하다 bad breath : 구취

3. 다음 영어의 뜻을 우리말로 쓰세요.

① I'd like to ask you some questions.

② I'm in poor health.

③ Are you pregnant?

④ Have you ever had any trouble with bleeding?

⑤ Are you receiving medical treatment now?

⑥ Have you ever had an anesthetic?

☞ in poor (good) health : 몸 상태가 안 좋다(건강하다)　pregnant:임신을 하고 있는　trouble : 곤란한 문제
receive : 받다, 경험하다　medical treatment : 치료　anesthetic : 마취제

4. 빈 칸에 "have, do, are"를 넣어 문장을 완성하세요.

① (　　　　) you taking any medicines?

② (　　　　) you have any allergies?

③ (　　　　) you allergic to any medication?

④ (　　　　) you ever had any serious illnesses?

⑤ (　　　　) you receiving medical treatment?

⑥ (　　　　) you pregnant?

⑦ (　　　　) you in good health?

⑧ (　　　　) you feel sick?

⑨ (　　　　) you suffering from hypertension?

☞ suffer from : (질병 등을) 앓다　hypertension : 고혈압

5. 치과위생사와 환자의 역할을 서로 정하세요. 치과위생사의 역할을 맡은 사람은 다음 문진표의 내용을 영어로 표현하고, 환자의 역할을 맡은 사람은 그 질문에 대답하세요.

병　력

성명

1. 건강상태가 좋습니까?	네,	아니요
2. 현재 무슨 치료를 받고 있습니까?	네,	아니요
3. 복용하고 계신 약이 있나요?	네,	아니요
4. 지금까지 심각한 병을 앓은 적이 있습니까?	네,	아니요
5. 지금까지 수술을 받은 적이 있습니까?	네,	아니요
6. 임신했습니까?	네,	아니요

Answer Key

1 ② met ③ eaten ④ visited ⑤ seen ⑥ written ⑦ lost

2 ① Have you ever had an operation? ② Have you ever had a dental checkup?
③ Have you ever been sick during dental treatment?
④ Have you ever cared about your bad breath?
⑤ Have you ever been here?

3 ① 질문이 있습니다. ② 저는 건강이 좋지 않습니다.
③ 임신하셨나요? ④ 출혈에 무슨 문제가 있습니까?
⑤ 요즈음 치료를 받고 있습니까? ⑥ 마취한 적이 있습니까?

4 ① Are ② Do ③ Are ④ Have ⑤ Are ⑥ Are ⑦ Are ⑧ Do ⑨ Are

UNIT 10 FOCUS

have+과거분사의 형태에는 두 가지 뜻이 있습니다.

① 계속　(unit 9)

시간이 흐르는 동안 계속되고 있습니다. 「계속 …하다」

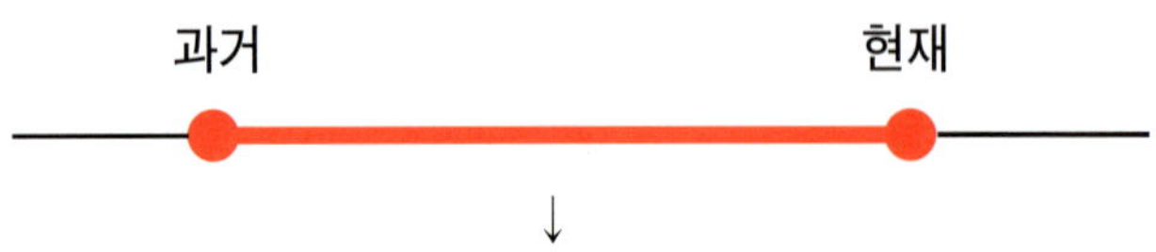

I have had a toothache for two days. (이틀 동안 이가 계속 아픕니다.)

② 경험　(unit 10)

시간이 흐르는 동안 경험한 적이 있습니다. 「…한 적이 있다」

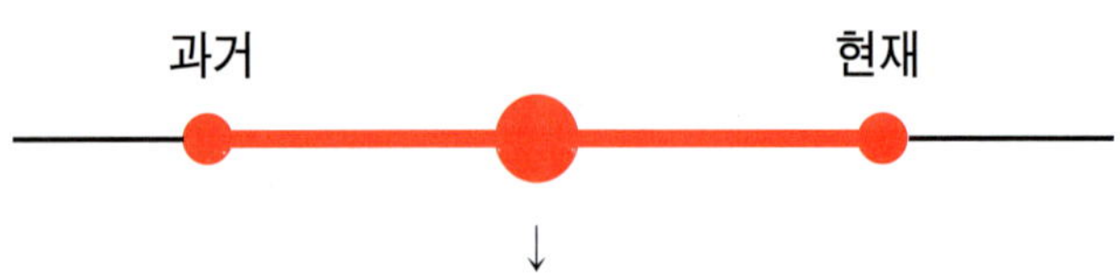

I have had a serious illness once. (저는 중병을 앓은 적이 한 번 있습니다.)

두 가지 모두 「시간이 흐르고 있다」는 공통점이 있습니다.

Exercise

1. 당신은 (1)~(3)을 한 적이 있습니까?
 다음의 예를 참고하여 「몇 번 ~한 적이 있다」라고 대답하세요.

(1) Have you ever been to a foreign country?

(2) Have you ever traveled alone?

(3) Have you ever written a letter in English?

(예)	I have never flown in an airplane.	(전혀 없다.)
	I have flown in an airplane once.	(한 번)
	I have flown in an airplane twice.	(두 번)
	I have flown in an airplane three times.	(세 번)

세 번 이상은 four times, six times처럼 number + times로 표현합니다.

2. 상대에게 (1)~(10)을 질문하고, YES라고 대답한 사람의 이름을 써 보세요.
 이름 쓰는 칸이 모두 채워질 때까지 여러 사람에게 질문해 보세요.

QUESTIONS	NAME
(1) Have you ever owned a pet?	
(2) Have you ever had a part-time job?	
(3) Have you ever ridden a jet coaster?	
(4) Have you ever gone skiing?	
(5) Have you ever gone fishing?	
(6) Have you ever visited Seoul?	
(7) Have you ever had a party with your friends?	
(8) Have you ever given a present to your parents?	
(9) Have you ever baked a cake?	
(10) Have you ever eaten Korean food?	

UNIT 11 Come this way, please.

Vocabulary

put on …을 입다, 몸에 달다, 쓰다, 신다 ⇔ *take off* (옷 · 모자 · 신발을) 벗다, 풀다

turn (… 쪽을) 향하다

bite (…를) 깨물다

rinse (입을) 헹구다

keep (어떤 상태를) 계속하다 — keep still : 가만히 있다

…을 (어떤 상태로) 유지하다 — keep your mouth open : 입을 계속 벌리다

1. 네모 속의 단어를 알맞은 형태로 바꾸어 빈 칸에 써 보세요.

keep	keep	rinse	take	put	bite	turn

① She _________ on her shoes and went out. (그녀는 신발을 신고 밖으로 나왔다.)

② I _________ off my glasses before going to bed. (나는 자기 전에 안경을 벗는다)

③ I _________ my teeth clean.(나는 치아를 깨끗이 유지한다.)

④ The girl _________ quiet.(그녀는 조용히 있었다.)

⑤ I _________ my mouth after eating.(나는 밥을 먹은 후에 입을 헹군다.)

⑥ She _________ her back to me. (그녀는 나에게 등을 돌렸다.)

⑦ When I _________ down a piece of ice, I felt pain.(얼음을 깨물었을 때 통증을 느꼈다.)

☞ when : …할 때에

Key sentences

Come this way, please. (이쪽으로 오시겠어요.)

Sit in this chair. (이 의자에 앉으세요.)

Please wait a while. (잠시만 기다려 주세요.)

Please open your mouth. (입을 벌려 주세요.)

Close your eyes. (눈을 감아 주세요.)

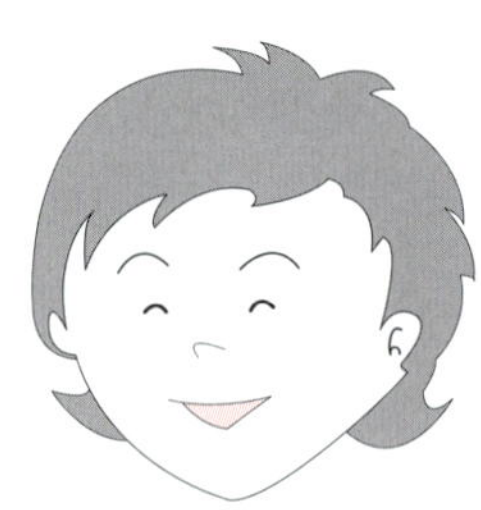

Relax. (편하게 계세요.)

Grammar & Speaking

주어 "you"를 생략하고 동사 원형으로 시작하는 문장을 명령문이라고 합니다. 명령문은 지시나 의뢰를 할 때 사용합니다. 문장의 앞이나 뒤에 "please"를 붙이면 정중한 표현입니다.

Come this way. ⇒ Please come this way. = Come this way, please.

명령문 앞에 "don't"를 붙이면 금지나 충고를 나타냅니다.

Please don' t smoke here.
(이곳에서는 담배를 필 수 없습니다.)

Please don't be late.	늦지 마세요.
swallow.	삼키지 마세요.
eat and drink for about an hour.	약 한 시간 동안은 금식하세요.
touch this part.	이 부분은 만지지 마세요.
close your mouth.	입을 다물지 마세요.
worry.	걱정하지 마세요.

Practice

2. ①~⑧의 그림을 나타내는 문장을 아래에서 고르세요.

①
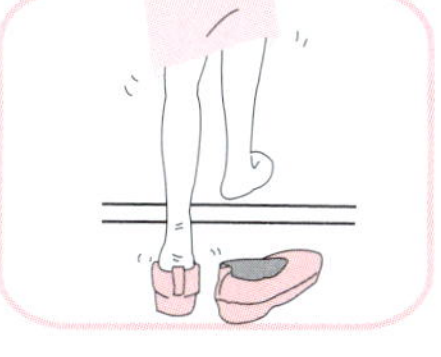
②
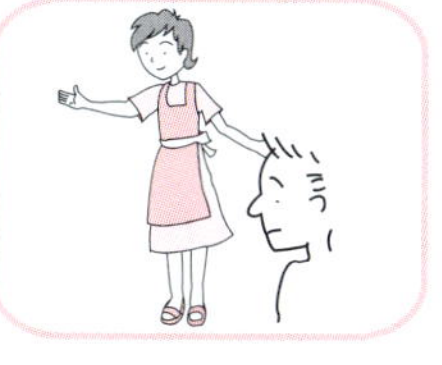
③
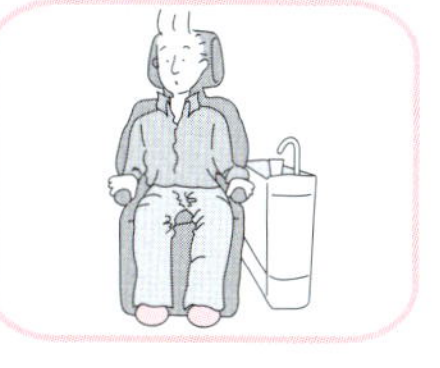
④
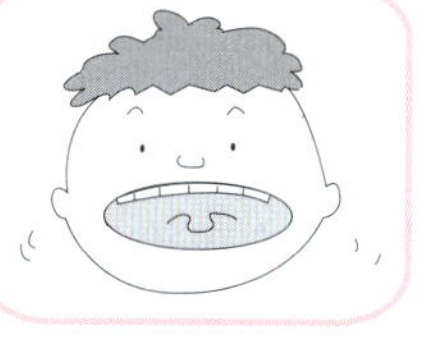
⑤
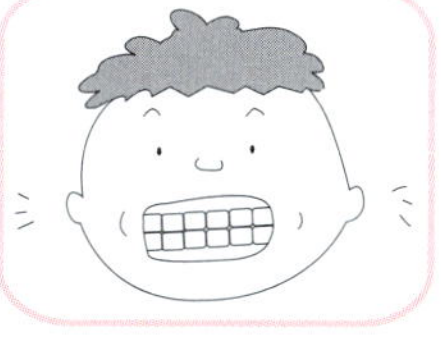
⑥
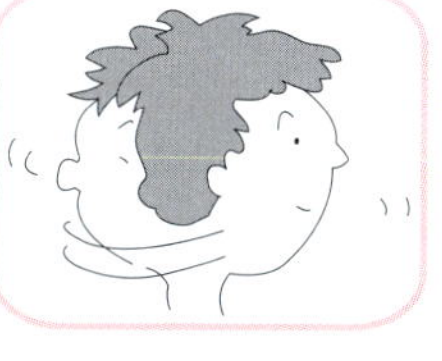
⑦
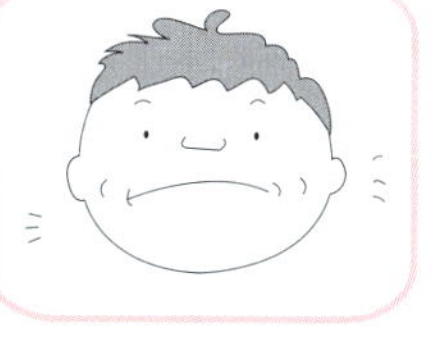
⑧
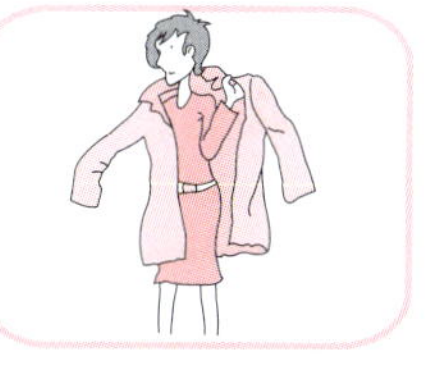

( ) Put on your coat.
( ) Take off your shoes.
( ) Close your mouth.
( ) Turn your head to the left.
( ) Come this way.
( ) Please bite down.
( ) Open your mouth wide.
( ) Sit in this chair.

3. 네모 속의 단어를 골라 빈 칸에 넣어서 영문을 작성하세요.

①~⑥

take	come	open	wait	put	keep

① Please (   ) in. (들어오세요.)

② Please (   ) off your shoes. (신발을 벗으세요.)

③ Please (   ) on the mules. (슬리퍼를 신으세요.)

☞ mules : 슬리퍼

④ (   ) here, please. (여기에서 기다리세요.)

⑤ (   ) your mouth wide. (입을 크게 벌려주세요.)

⑥ (   ) your teeth together. (입을 다물고 계세요.)

⑦~⑫

be	turn	take	rinse	keep	bite

⑦ (   ) your head to the right. (오른쪽으로 돌리세요.)

⑧ (   ) this cotton roll. (솜을 꽉 무세요.)

⑨ Please (   ) still. (가만히 계세요.)

⑩ (   ) your mouth. (입을 헹구세요.)

⑪ (   ) careful. (조심하세요.)

⑫ (   ) care of yourself. (조심하세요.)

☞ careful : (…에) 주의 깊은　　take care of : 조심하다

4. 왼쪽의 단어와 이에 맞는 구절을 선으로 연결하세요.

① come ·	· your mouth wide / your eyes / your book to page 10
② sit ·	· still / your mouth open / your teeth together
③ wait ·	· this way / in / with me
④ close ·	· your shoes / your coat / your glasses
⑤ open ·	· a while / a minute / here
⑥ put on ·	· your head to the left / your back to me
⑦ rinse ·	· in this chair / down / at the table
⑧ turn ·	· your eyes / your mouth / the window
⑨ keep ·	· your mouth / the dishes / the shirts

5. 빈 칸에 알맞은 단어를 쓰세요.

① Excuse me, but please (　　　　) off your shoes.

② Please have a seat and (　　　　) a while.

③ (　　　　) this way.

④ Please (　　　　) in this chair.

⑤ Please (　　　　) on this apron.

⑥ (　　　　) your mouth wide.

⑦ (　　　　) your head to the right.

⑧ (　　　　) down.

⑨ (　　　　) your mouth with the mouthwash.

⑩ (　　　　) your teeth clean.

☞ have a seat : 앉다　　apron : 앞치마　　mouthwash : 구강세정액

6. 다음의 내용을 영어로 표현하세요.

1. 환자를 진료실 의자로 안내하세요.

2. 환자에게 다음의 내용을 지시하세요.

① 입을 벌려 주세요.

② 입을 다물어 주세요.

③ 편하게 계세요.

④ 아프면(If you feel pain,) 오른 손을 들어 주세요.

⑤ 조심하세요.

Answer Key

1 ① put ② take ③ keep ④ kept ⑤ rinse ⑥ turned ⑦ bit

2 ① Take off your shoes. ② Come this way. ③ Sit in this chair. ④ Open your mouth wide. ⑤ Please bite down. ⑥ Turn your head to the left. ⑦ Close your mouth. ⑧ Put on your coat.

3 ① come ② take ③ put ④ wait ⑤ open ⑥ keep ⑦ turn ⑧ bite ⑨ keep ⑩ rinse ⑪ be ⑫ take

4 ① come this way / in / with me ② sit in(on) this chair / down / at the table
③ wait a while / a minute / here ④ close your eyes / your mouth / the window
⑤ open your mouth wide / your eyes / your book to page 10
⑥ put on your shoes / your coat / your glasses ⑦ rinse your mouth / the dishes / the shirts
⑧ turn your head to the left / your back to me ⑨ keep still / your mouth open / your teeth together

5 ① take ② wait ③ come ④ sit ⑤ put ⑥ open ⑦ turn ⑧ bite ⑨ rinse ⑩ keep

6 예 1. I'm sorry to have kept you waiting. : (기다리시게 하여 죄송합니다.)
Come this way, please. Sit in this chair. Please wait a while.
2. ① Keep your mouth open (,please). ② Close your mouth (,please).
③ Relax(,please). ④ If you feel pain, raise your right hand.
⑤ Take (good) care of yourself.

UNIT 11 FOCUS

명령문을 사용하여 길을 안내할 수 있습니다. 지시의 기본표현을 배워봅시다.

〈지시〉

Go straight. (똑바로 가세요.)

Turn right (left). (오른쪽(왼쪽)으로 돌아가세요.)

Turn right (left) at the first corner. (첫 모퉁이에서 오른쪽으로(왼쪽으로) 돌아가세요.)

〈장소를 표현하는 방법〉

A is next to B. (A는 B 옆에 있습니다.)

A is between B and C. (A는 B와 C 사이에 있습니다.)

A is on the right (left). (A는 오른쪽(왼쪽)에 있습니다.)

A is across from D. (A는 D의 맞은편에 있습니다.)

E is on the corner. (E는 모퉁이에 있습니다.)

F is on the 3rd floor. (F는 3층에 있습니다.)

MAP

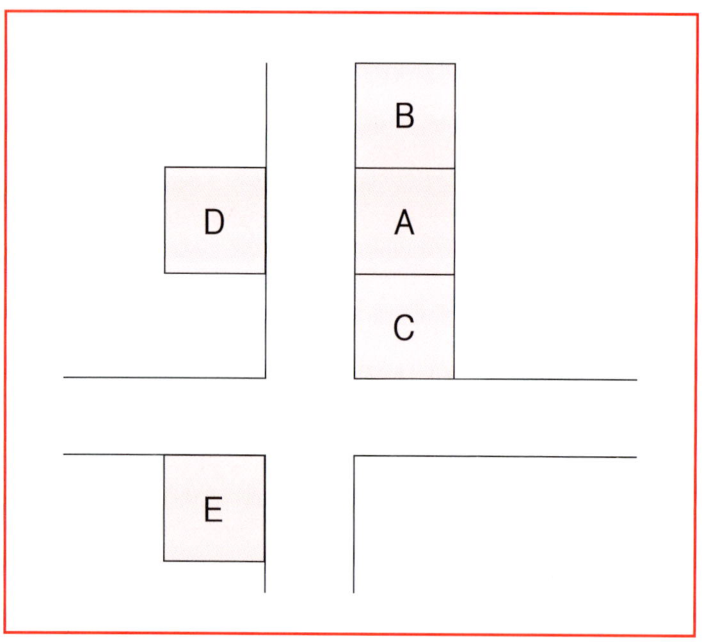

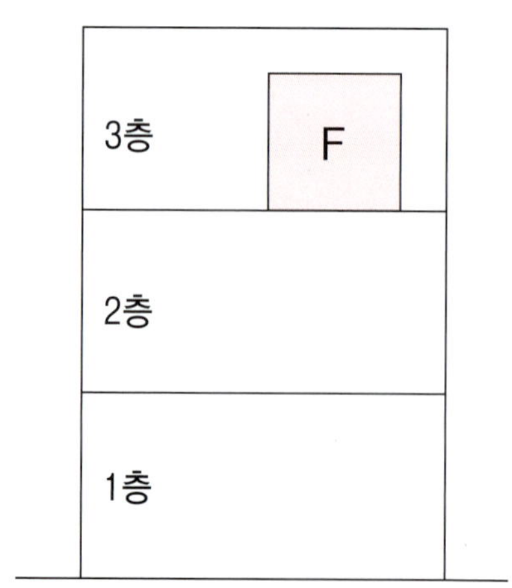

Exercise

1. 실제로 길 안내를 해보세요. 아래 그림은 근처 역에서 치과의원까지 오는 약도입니다. 역에서 오는 길을 안내해 보세요.

MAP

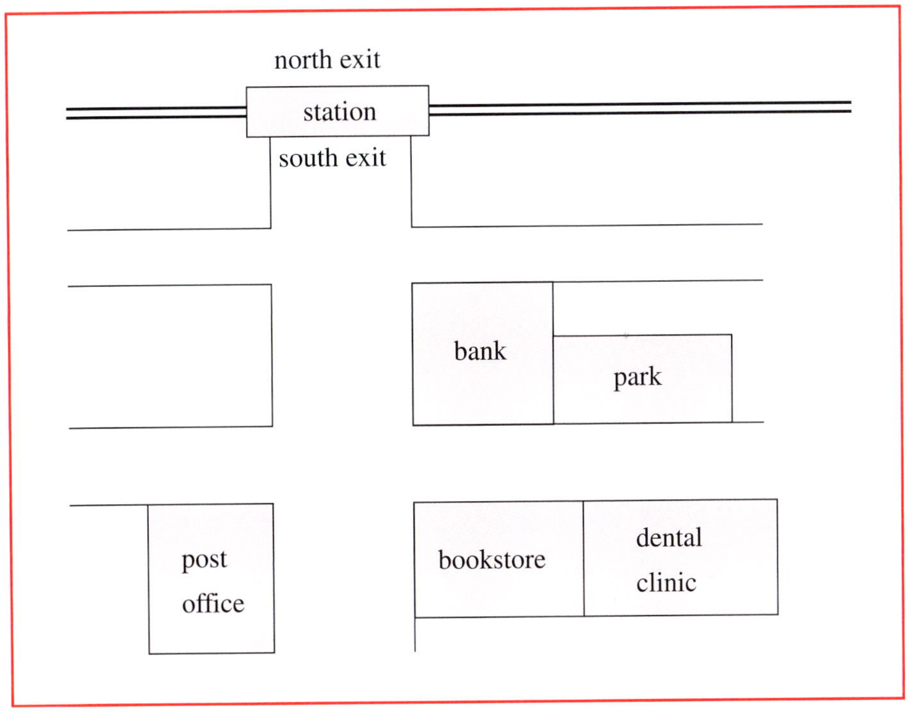

(길의 순서)

(1)

(2)

(3)

Answer Key

(1) Please leave the station by the south exit.

(2) Go straight and turn left at the second corner.

(3) The dental clinic is on your right.

The dental clinic is next to the bookstore.

The dental clinic is just past the bookstore.

The dental clinic is across from the park.

UNIT 12 The doctor will take some X-rays of your teeth.

Vocabulary

take	(사진을) 찍다
take out	(…을) 꺼내다
put	(어느 장소에) 두다
hold	(손으로) 잡다
recline	(의자를) 뒤로 젖히다
sit	(…에) 앉다

①
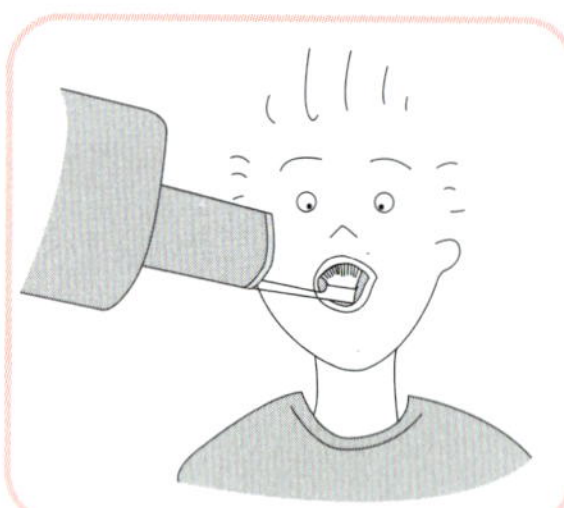
take an X-ray

②
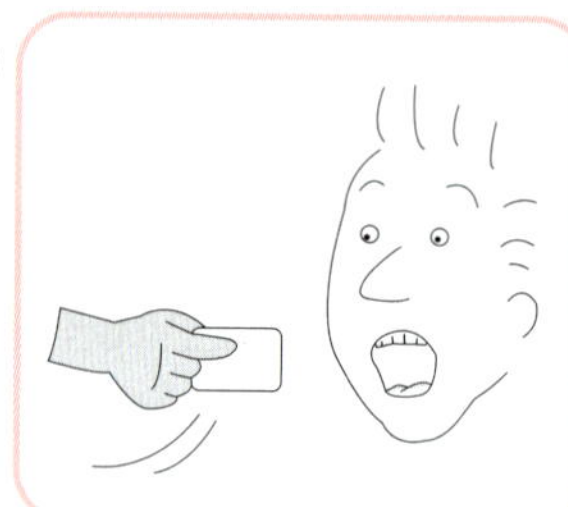
put a film in your mouth

③
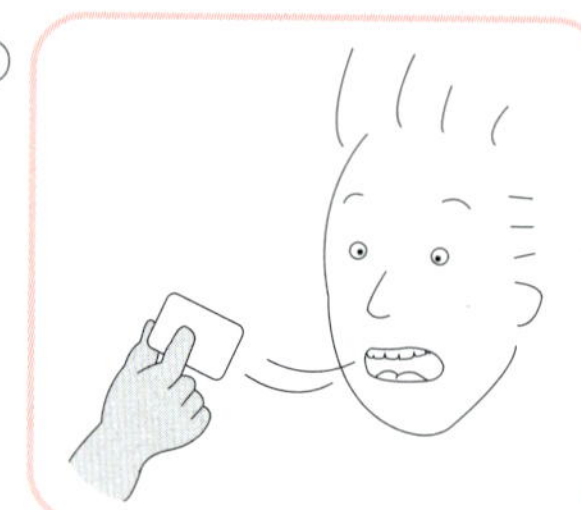
take out a film from your mouth

④
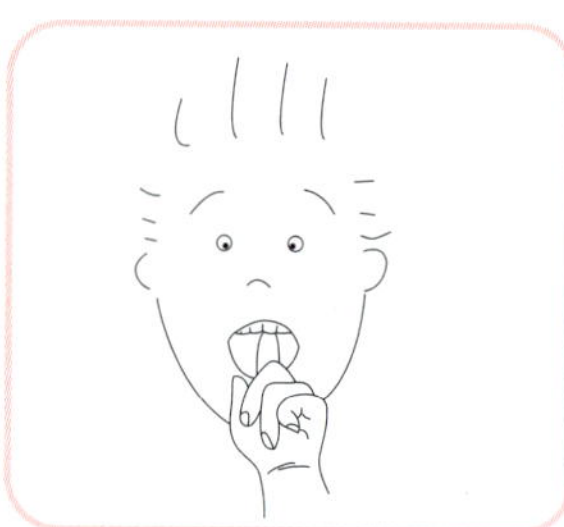
hold a film with your finger

⑤
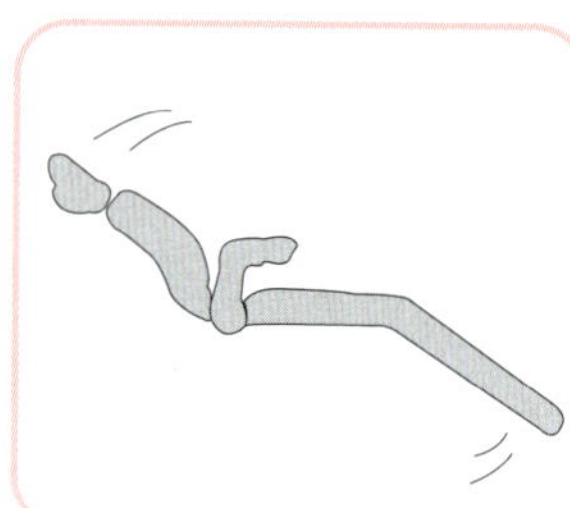
recline the seat

⑥
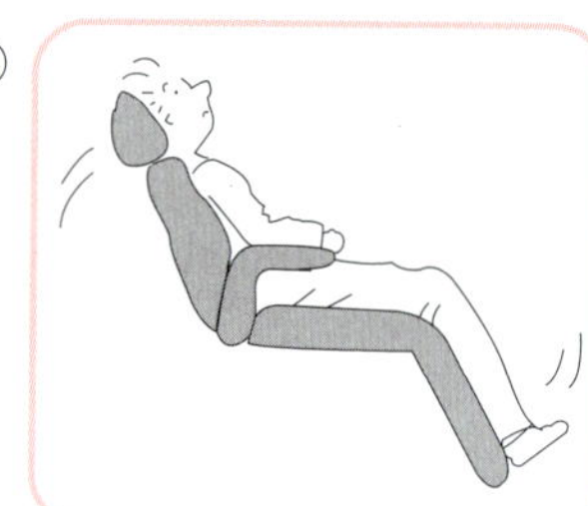
sit you up

☞ ① X선 사진을 찍다. ② 입에 필름을 넣다. ③ 필름을 꺼내다.
④ 손가락으로 필름을 누르다. ⑤ 의자를 뒤로 눕히다. ⑥ (사람을) 일으켜 세우다.

1. 왼쪽 단어에 맞는 구절을 선으로 연결하세요.

take ·	1) a key on the table / a filling in your tooth / some milk in my coffee
put ·	2) you up / the child at the table / down
hold ·	3) an X-ray / an impression of your mouth / your picture
sit ·	4) the bag / a baby in my arms / a film with your finger
take ·	5) out a bad tooth / out a cotton roll from your mouth

☞ impression : 인상 picture : 사진 firmly : 확실하게

Key sentences

The doctor will take some X-rays of your teeth. Please wait here.
(의사선생님께서 치아의 X선 사진을 찍으실 겁니다.) (여기에서 기다려 주세요.)

Open your mouth. I'll put a film in your mouth.
(입을 벌리세요.) (제가 필름을 입에 넣겠습니다.)

Please hold the film with your fingers. Keep still.
(손가락으로 필름을 눌러 주세요.) (가만히 계세요.)

I'll take out the film. (필름을 꺼내겠습니다.)

I'll recline the chair. (의자를 뒤로 눕히겠습니다.)

I'll sit you up. (의자를 세우겠습니다.)

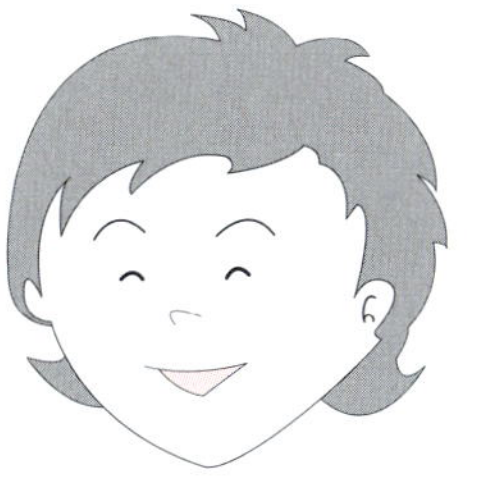

☞ I'll = I will

Grammar

will (1) …일 것이다, …이겠지 (2) …라고 생각한다, …할 생각이다

영어의 미래 시제는 <will>을 사용하여 표현할 수 있습니다. <will>은 (1) 단순하게 미래를 나타내거나 (2) 「…할 생각이다」 등의 의사를 표현합니다.

(1) 단순히 미래를 나타내는 <will> (…일 것이다, …이겠지)

1. I missed the train. I'll be late. (기차를 놓쳤다. 늦을 것 같다.)
2. Don't eat too much candy. You'll have a toothache. (사탕을 너무 많이 먹지 마세요. 치통이 생길지 모릅니다.)

(2) 의사를 나타내는 <will> (……라고 생각한다, …할 생각이다)

3. It's a nice day. I'll go for a walk. (날씨가 좋다. 산책을 해야겠다.)
4. You look so busy. I'll help you. (바쁜 것 같군요. 제가 도와 드릴게요.)

☞ 단축형 I'll = I will you'll = you will he'll = he will she'll = she will it'll = it will
we'll = we will they'll = they will won't = will not

2. ①~④에 이어지는 문장을 A~D에서 선택하세요. <will: 미래>

① I'd like to talk to Dr. Kim. (　　　　　)

② I don't feel very well. (　　　　　)

③ May I call you tonight? (　　　　　)

④ My son fell down the stairs and hit his head. (　　　　　)

A. Take him to the hospital. He'll have some X-rays.

B. Yes. I'll be home tonight.

C. Go home and sleep well. You'll feel better tomorrow.

D. I'm afraid he is out. He'll be back in ten minutes.

☞ fell : fall (떨어지다)의 과거형　fall down : 떨어지다　take : (…으로) 데리고 가다

① 김 선생님과 말씀을 나누고 싶습니다. ② 기분이 별로 좋지 않습니다.

③ 오늘 밤에 전화를 드려도 될까요?　④ 제 아들이 계단에서 떨어져 머리를 부딪쳤습니다.

A. 아들을 병원으로 데리고 가세요. X선 사진을 찍어야 할 것 같습니다.

B: 네, 오늘 밤은 집에 있을 겁니다.

C. 집에 가서 푹 주무세요. 내일이면 더 좋아지실 겁니다.

D. 선생님은 외출하셨는데요. 10분 안에 돌아오실 겁니다.

3. [ ]의 단어를 골라 빈 칸에 넣어 문장을 완성하세요. <will: 의지>

〔 put　hold　clean　show　take 〕

① I'll (　　　　) your coat in the basket. Take out your valuables from the pockets.

② Do you have an insurance card?　Yes, I'll (　　　　) you.

③ Please open your mouth. I'll (　　　　) out the cotton roll.

④ Please take out your dentures. I'll (　　　　) them for you.

⑤ I'll (　　　　) this mirror. Check your brushing.

☞ valuables : 귀중품　liquid : 액체

① 코트를 옷장에 넣어 드리겠습니다. 주머니에서 귀중품을 꺼내세요.　② 보험증은 갖고 계신가요? 네, 여기 있습니다.

③ 입을 벌려 주세요. 솜을 꺼내겠습니다.　④ 의치를 빼 주세요. 의치를 깨끗이 청소해 드리겠습니다.

⑤ 제가 거울을 들고 있겠습니다. 이를 잘 닦았는지 확인하세요.

Answer Key

1 take — 3), put — 1), hold — 4), sit — 2), take — 5)

2 1 — D 2 — C 3 — B 4 — A

3 1 — put 2 — show 3 — take 4 — clean 5 — hold

UNIT 12 FOCUS

지금까지 공부한 시간의 표현을 복습해 봅시다.

과거	현재	미래
↓	↓	↓
① 과거형	② 현재형	③ will
You were busy (yesterday).	You are busy.	You'll be busy (tomorrow).
She was here.	She is here.	She'll be here.
She liked "natto".	She likes "natto".	She'll like "natto".
He had lunch there.	He has lunch there.	He'll have lunch there.

동사의 형태에 주의!

① 과거형은 -ed를 붙이는 경우가 많습니다. 하지만 예외(불규칙형)도 있으므로 사전을 찾아 공부하세요.

② 현재형은 기본형입니다. 하지만 예외로 「나와 당신이 아닌 제삼자」는 (He/She/It)에 -s를 붙이는 것을 기억하세요.

③ 미래형은 will+ 동사입니다. will 뒤에는 -ed, -s를 붙이지 않습니다.

× She will is there. → ◯ She will be there.

× He will washed dishes in the kitchen. → ◯ He will wash dishes in the kitchen.

× He will has lunch there. → ◯ He will have lunch there.

Exercise

과거, 현재, 미래에 관하여 (1)~(7)의 영어 질문에 대답하세요.
동사형에 주의하세요.

(1) Where did you grow up?

(2) When you were a child, which did you like better, reading books or playing outside?

(3) What kind of games did you like?

(4) What kind of dreams did you have?

(5) Where do you live now? Do you like there?

(6) Which subject do you like best? Why do you like it?

(7) Who do you respect? Why do you respect him/her?

(8) What do you want to be?

(9) Where will you live in the future?

(10) What kind of life will you live?

UNIT 13 Take one tablet three times a day.

Vocabulary

<medicine>

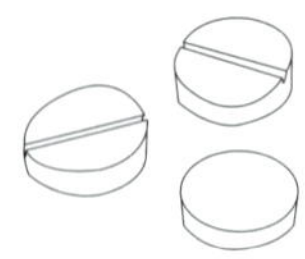

tablet 알약(정제)

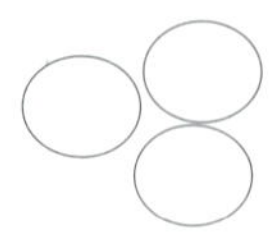

pill 환약

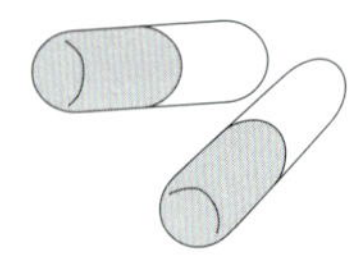

capsule 캡슐

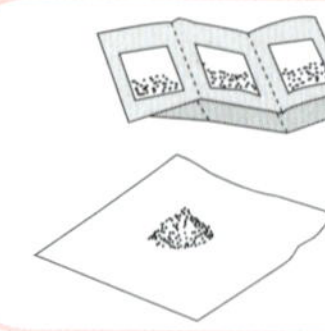

powder 가루약

mouthwash	구강세정액, 입을 헹구는 약		
antibiotics	항생제		
injection	주사	give an injection	주사를 놓다
		have an injection	주사를 맞다
anesthetic	마취제	a local anesthetic	국소마취

painkiller : 진통제

prescription : 처방전

Key sentences

Here is your medicine. (당신 약입니다.)

These are antibiotics. (항생제입니다)

Take one tablet 3 times a day. (하루에 한 알씩 세 번 복용하세요)

How often do I take this medicine? (이 약은 몇 번 먹습니까?)

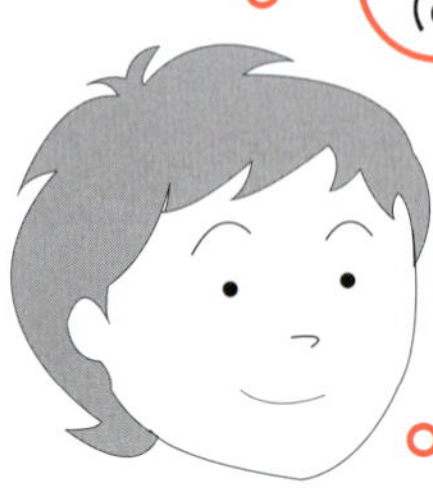

When do I take? (언제 먹습니까?)

After meals. (식사 후에 먹습니다.)

How many days do I take this medicine ? (이 약은 며칠 동안 먹나요?)

For 3 days. (사흘 동안입니다)

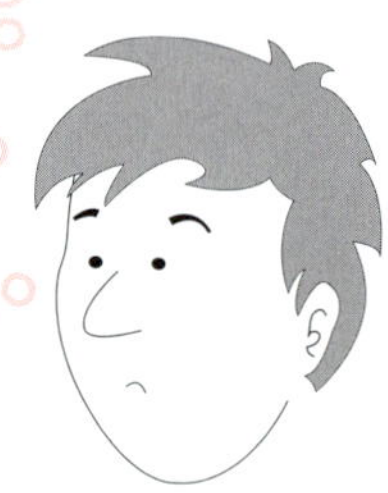

Take one tablet 3 times a day after meals for 3 days. (하루 세 번 식후에 한 알씩 사흘 동안 복용하세요)

These are painkillers. (이것은 진통제입니다)

Take one tablet when you have pain. (통증이 있을 때 한 알씩 드세요)

☞ here : 이쪽으로, 여기에

1. 네모 속의 단어를 골라 빈 칸에 넣어 문장을 완성하세요.

cavity	take	injection	toothache	medicine	anesthetic	filling

I had a terrible ( ), so I went to the dentist. She examined my teeth and found a ( ). She said, "It needs a ( ). I'll use a local ( ) before drilling. Are you allergic to an anesthetic?" I said, "No, I'm not." Then I had an ( ). The drilling was not painful. After treatment, she gave me ( ) and said, "These are pain-killers. ( ) one tablet when you have pain."

☞ suffer from : (질병을) 앓다　　hypertension : 고혈압

2. 네모 속의 구절을 골라 빈 칸에 넣어 영문을 작성하세요.

Take one tablet ( ). 식후에 한 알(정)씩 드세요.

Take one tablet ( ). 식전에 한 알씩 드세요.

Take one tablet ( ). 아침과 저녁식사 후에 한 알씩 드세요.

Take one tablet ( ). 식사 사이에 한 알씩 드세요.

Take one tablet ( ). 잠자기 전에 한 알씩 드세요.

Take one tablet ( ). 하루에 한 번 한 알씩 드세요.

Take one tablet ( ). 하루에 두 번 한 알씩 드세요.

Take one tablet ( ). 여덟 시간마다 한 알씩 드세요.

Take one tablet ( ). 닷새 동안 한 알씩 드세요.

Take this ( ). 의사의 지시에 따라 약을 드세요.

before meals / once a day / after meals / for 5 days

between meals / every 8 hours / twice a day / before going to bed

after breakfast and dinner / following your doctor's instructions

3. 아래 영문의 빈 칸을 채우고, 약봉지에 쓰여 있는 약의 복용법을 설명하세요.

내복약 ______________________ **님**			
	1일	3회	3일분
가루약은 1회			포
알약은 1회			정
캡슐은 1회		1개	
(아침)	식전	매시간	
(점심)	자기 전	식사 사이	
(저녁)	식후		
	의사의 지시에 따라		
	김 치과의원		

Here is your (   ) .

Take one capsule (   ) a day

(   ) meals.

Take these capsules (   ) 3 days.

4. 내복약 A와 B를 영어로 설명하세요.

[A]

내복약 ______________________ **님**			
	1일	2회	5일분
가루약은 1회			포
알약은 1회			1정
캡슐은 1회		개	
(아침)	식전	매시간	
점심	자기 전	식사 사이	
(저녁)	(식후)		
	의사의 지시에 따라		
	김 치과의원		

[B]

내복약 ______________________ **님**		
캡슐 1개는 8시간마다		
1회	1알	3일분
알약은 통증이 있을 때		
1회	1정	
정덴탈클리닉		

Answer Key

1 I had a terrible (toothache), so I went to the dentist. She examined my teeth and found a (cavity). She said, "It needs a (filling). I'll use a local (anesthetic) before drilling. Are you allergic to an anesthetic?" I said, "No, I'm not." Then I had an (injection). The drilling was not painful. After treatment, she gave me (medicine) and said, "These are pain-killers. (Take) one tablet when you have pain."

2 after meals (식후에) / before meals (식전에) / after breakfast and dinner (아침과 저녁식사 후에) / between meals (식사 사이에) / before going to bed (잠자기 전에) / once a day (하루 한 번) / twice a day (하루 두 번) / every 8 hours (여덟 시간마다) / for 5 days (닷새 동안) / following your doctor's instructions (의사의 지시에 따라)

3 medicine, 3 times, after, for

4 《예》

[A] Here is your medicine.
Take one tablet twice a day after breakfast and dinner for 5 days.

[B] There are two kinds of medicine in this bag.
Take one capsule every 8 hours for 3 days.
These tablets are painkillers. When you have pain, take one tablet.

UNIT 13 FOCUS

「당신이 드실 약입니다.」는 "Here is your medicine"이라고 합니다. 회화를 할 때 기억하면 편리한 표현이 많으므로 연습해 보세요.

(1)	No problem. My pleasure. You're welcome.	천만에요.
(2)	All right.	걱정하지 마세요. 괜찮습니다.
(3)	I'm sorry. That's too bad.	죄송합니다.
(4)	Just a minute.	잠시만 기다리세요.
(5)	How about you?	당신은 어떠세요?
(6)	Take your time.	천천히 하세요.
(7)	Watch your step ! Watch out!	위험해요! 조심하세요!
(8)	This medicine works well.	이 약은 잘 듣습니다.
(9)	Let me see... Well...	저….
(10)	Take care. You too.	몸조심하세요. 당신도요.
(12)	See you next week.	다음 주에 뵙겠습니다.

Exercise

1. 빈도를 나타내는 표현을 배워 봅시다.

빈도가 높다	(100%)	always
		usually
		often
		sometimes
		occasionally
		seldom (rarely)
빈도가 낮다	(0%)	never

2. 빈도에 관한 질문입니다. "How often do you…?"를 사용하여 상대에게 질문하세요.
   대답을 잘 듣고 표에 이름을 써보세요.

	everyday	often	sometimes	seldom	never
go to the movies					
work part-time					
go shopping					
read books					
watch TV					

UNIT 14 You should brush before bedtime.

Key sentences

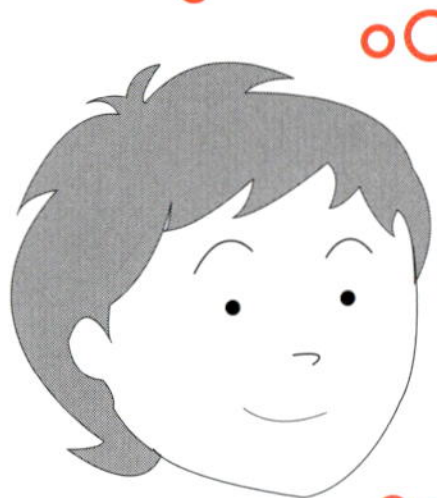

How many times a day do you brush your teeth?
(하루에 몇 번 이를 닦습니까?)

Once. (한 번이요.)

When do you brush?
(언제 닦습니까?)

After breakfast.
(아침식사 후에요.)

You should brush before bedtime.
(주무시기 전에 이를 닦아야 합니다.)

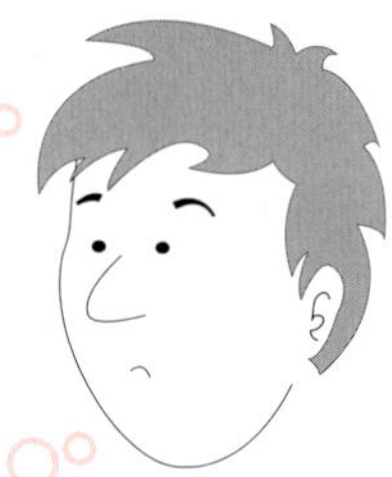

Brush at least 10 minutes.
(적어도 10분은 닦으세요.)

How long should I brush?
(얼마나 오래 닦아야 하나요?)

What kind of toothbrush do you use?
(어떤 종류의 칫솔을 사용하나요?)

A soft toothbrush.
(부드러운 칫솔을 사용합니다.)

☞ bedtime : 자는 시간

Grammar

should …하는 것이 좋다: …해야 한다

✐ You should do something = it is a good thing to do

You should brush at least once a day.	(적어도 하루에 한 번은 이를 닦아야 합니다)
You should take your time while brushing.	(천천히 시간을 두고 이를 닦아야 합니다)

✐ Should I brush after eating?	(식후에 이를 닦는 것이 좋습니까?)
Should I brush my tongue?	(혀도 닦는 것이 좋습니다)
How should I brush?	(어떻게 닦으면 되나요?)
When should I change my toothbrush?	(칫솔은 언제 바꿔야 하나요?)

✐ You shouldn't do something = it is not a good thing to do

You shouldn't scrub your teeth.	(이를 문질러 닦으면 안 됩니다)
You shouldn't brush your teeth too vigorously.	(이를 너무 세게 닦으면 안 됩니다.)

☞ take one's time : 천천히 하다　　scrub : 문지르다　　vigorously : 세게

1. 다음의 내용을 "should"를 사용하여 「하는 것이 좋다고 생각합니다.」와 「해서는 안 돼요.」로 나누어 보세요.

use a toothbrush with natural bristles (천연 모로 만든 칫솔을 사용한다.)

brush your tongue (혀를 칫솔로 닦는다.)

use a lot of toothpaste at every brushing (칫솔질을 할 때마다 치약을 많이 묻혀 사용한다.)

floss your teeth once a day (하루에 한 번씩 치실로 치아 사이를 닦는다.)

replace your toothbrush every 2 to 3 months (2~3개월마다 칫솔을 바꾼다.)

use a fluoride toothpaste (불소가 들어있는 치약을 사용한다.)

eat sugary snacks and sugary drinks (설탕이 들어간 과자나 단 음료수를 먹는다.)

use an electric toothbrush (전동칫솔을 사용한다.)

brush your teeth vigorously (강하게 힘을 주어 이를 닦는다.)

have a lot of soda (탄산음료수를 많이 마신다.)

☞ bristle : (칫솔)모 floss : (치아 사이를) 치실로 닦는다. fluoride toothpaste : 불소가 들어간 치약
sugary : 설탕이 들어있는, 단 electric : 전동의

You should do.

You shouldn't do.

How To Brush

To keep your teeth healthy, get into proper brushing.

- Brush at least once every day (It's important to brush before bedtime).
- Take your time brushing. You should spend at least 10 minutes.
- Replace your toothbrush when the bristles are spread.
- Use a fluoride toothpaste.

1. Bass Method

Be sure to use a toothbrush with soft bristles. Place bristles at a 45-degree angle where the teeth meet the gums. Gently brush the teeth using a vibrating back & forth motion. This method is effective for treatment and prevention of periodontal disease.

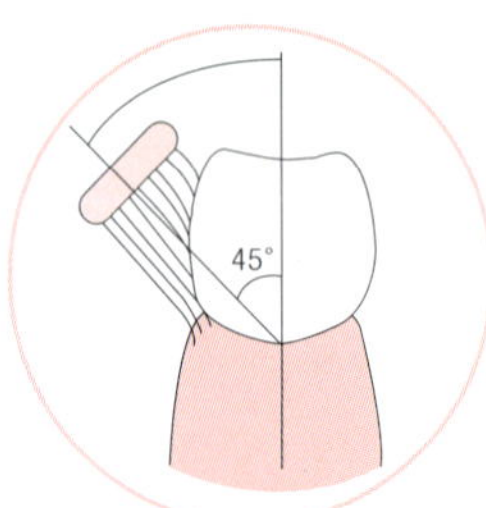

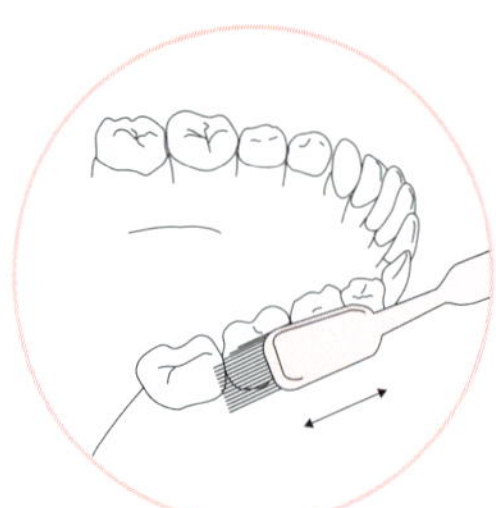

2. Scrubbing Method

Place bristles at a right angle to the teeth. Move the brush back & forth with a short stroke. Be careful not to use a long stroke.

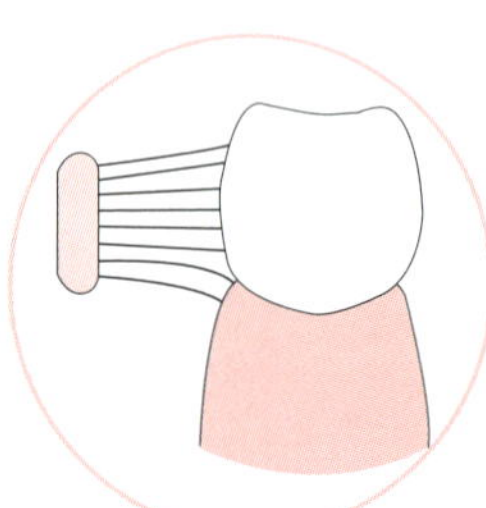

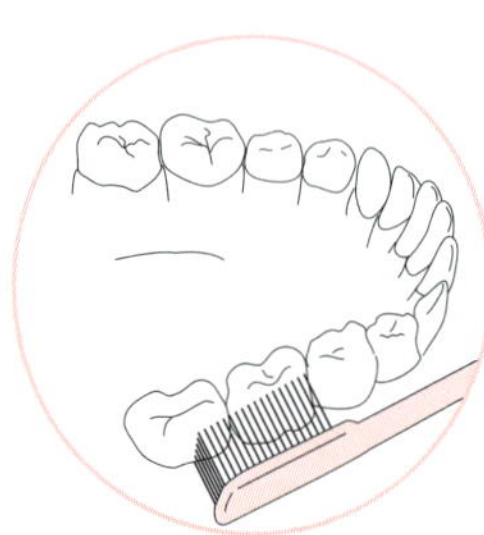

get into : (습관을) 익히다
spend : (시간을) 쓰다
a 45-degree angle : 45도
effective : 효과적인(효과가 큰)
prevention : 예방
stroke : 한 번의 동작
proper : 적절한
replace : (…)을 바꾸다
meet : 만나다
treatment : 치료(법)
periodontal disease : 치주질환(치주병)
a right angle : 직각

칫솔질 방법

치아 건강을 위해 정확한 칫솔질 방법을 배우도록 하세요.

적어도 하루 한 번씩은 이를 닦아야 합니다. (자기 전에 이를 닦는 것이 중요합니다).

천천히 양치질을 합니다. 적어도 십분 정도는 닦아야 합니다.

칫솔모가 구부러지면 칫솔을 바꾸세요.

불소가 들어있는 치약을 사용하세요.

1. 바스법

칫솔은 반드시 칫솔모가 부드러운 제품을 사용하세요. 치아가 잇몸과 만나는 곳에 칫솔을 45도 각도로 위치합니다. 칫솔을 앞뒤로 움직여 진동을 주면서 치아를 부드럽게 닦습니다. 치주질환의 치료나 예방에 효과적인 칫솔질 방법입니다.

2. 횡마법

칫솔모를 치아에 직각으로 대고, 앞뒤로 짧은 동작을 주어 칫솔을 움직입니다. 칫솔을 큰 동작으로 움직이지 않도록 주의하세요.

Practice

2. ①~⑤에 이어지는 구절을 오른쪽에서 고르세요.

① take	· a fluoride toothpaste
② brush	· your toothbrush when the bristles are spread
③ replace	· your time
④ floss	· your teeth (to clean between your teeth)
⑤ use	· your teeth gently

3. 아래에서 단어를 골라 빈 칸에 넣어 문장을 완성하세요.

How many　　Where　　How　　What　　How long　　When

① (　　　) kind of toothbrush do you use?	A hard toothbrush.
② (　　　) times a day should I brush?	At least once a day.
③ (　　　) do you brush your teeth?	After eating.
④ (　　　) do you brush?	For 2 or 3 minutes.
⑤ (　　　) does it hurt?	Some of my lower teeth.
⑥ (　　　) do you go to work?	By train.

Answer Key

2 ① your time ② your teeth gently ③ your toothbrush when the bristles are spread ④ your teeth (to clean between your teeth) ⑤ a fluoride toothpaste

3 ① What ② How many ③ When ④ How long ⑤ Where ⑥ How

부사(-ly가 붙어있는 단어)를 사용하면 동사를 더 자세히 설명할 수 있습니다.

Brush your teeth softly.

Please read the textbook carefully.

Could you speak slowly?

Please move quietly.

Exercise

조동사를 사용하면 정중한 표현을 할 수 있습니다.
각 표현의 역할을 확인하세요.

《자신의 요구를 정중하게 표현한다.》

I want to have a cup of tea. → I would like to have a cup of tea.
May I have a cup of tea?

《정중하게 지시한다.》

Come here. → I would like you to come here.
Can you come here?
Will you come here?
Would you come here?

(　　)의 조동사를 써서 다음의 표현을 바꿔 보세요.

1. I want to see Dr. Chung. (would를 사용하여 정중하게 표현한다)

2. Tell me how to brush my teeth. (will을 사용하여 정중하게 부탁한다)

3. Take off your shoes. (would를 사용하여 정중하게 부탁한다)

Answer Key

1. I want to see Dr. Chung.
2. Will you tell me how to brush my teeth?
3. Would you take off your shoes?

UNIT 15 Tartar should be removed by the dental hygienist.

Vocabulary

① *plaque* 치면세균막 — plaque control 치면세균막 관리

② *tartar* (*dental calculus*) 치석

③ *stain* 착색

④ *cause* …의 원인이다

⑤ *remove* 제거하다

Key sentences

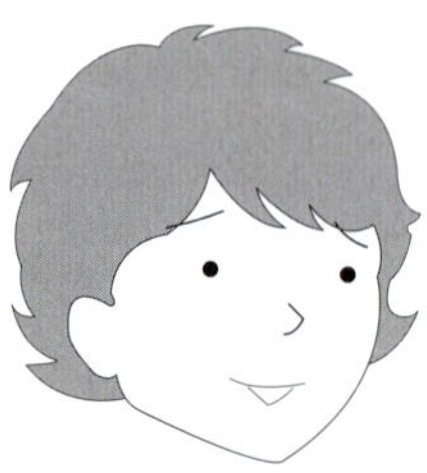

You have a lot of tartar on your teeth.
(치아에 치석이 많이 쌓여 있습니다.)

You can't remove tartar by brushing.
치석은 칫솔질로 제거할 수 없습니다.

Tartar should be removed by the dental hygienist.
치석은 치과위생사가 제거하는 것이 좋습니다.

Grammar & Speaking

be + done …된다

〈be+과거분사〉이고, 주어가 어떤 동작을 다른 사람에게 받는 수동태가 됩니다.

The car is washed by us every day.

(나는 매일 세차를 합니다)

We wash the car every day.

수동태는 be가 바뀌어 시제가 달라집니다. 조동사를 사용한 문장은 〈조동사+be+과거분사〉의 형태로 문장을 만듭니다.

The car was washed by us. (=We washed the car.) (우리는 세차를 했습니다.)

The car will be washed by us. (=We will wash the car.) (우리는 세차를 할 것입니다.)

The car is being washed by us. (=We are washing the car.) (우리는 세차를 하고 있습니다.)

The car has been washed by us. (=We have washed the car.) (우리는 세차를 한 적이 있습니다.)

The car should be washed by us. (=We should wash the car.) (우리는 세차를 해야 합니다.)

◇ 수동태의 문장을 소리 내어 연습해 보세요.

I was taken to the hospital by ambulance.	(나는 응급차에 실려 병원에 갔습니다.)
I was hit on the head.	(내 머리를 부딪쳤습니다.)
One of my front teeth is broken.	(저의 앞니 가운데 하나가 깨졌습니다.)
Plaque is removed by proper brushing.	(칫솔질을 제대로 하면 치면세균막을 제거할 수 있습니다.)
The tartar was removed by the dental hygienists.	(치과위생사가 치석을 제거해 주었습니다.)
Stains on your teeth are caused by tobacco.	(당신 치아의 착색은 담배가 원인입니다.)
The gums are swollen. It is called gingivitis.	(잇몸이 부었습니다.) (이를 치은염이라고 합니다.)

Practice

1. 다음의 문장을 밑줄 친 부분이 주어가 되는 수동태로 바꾸세요.

① We clean the clinic every day. (우리는 치과의원을 매일 청소합니다.)

② She took me to the station. (그녀가 나를 역으로 데려다 주었습니다.)

③ The dentist removed the tartar. (치과의사가 치석을 제거했습니다.)

④ Smoking will damage your health. (흡연은 건강을 해칩니다.)

2. 네모 속의 단어를 올바른 형태로 바꾸어 빈 칸에 넣어 수동태의 문장을 만드세요.

use	cause	damage	remove	call	~~hit~~

① I was (hit) in the face.

② Your teeth will be ( ) by eating too much candy.

③ Floss is ( ) to clean between teeth.

④ Your name will soon be ( ) .

⑤ Lipstick was ( ) with a tissue.

⑥ Tooth staining can be ( ) by coffee or tea.

☞ ① 내 얼굴을 맞았다. ② 사탕을 너무 많이 먹으면 이가 상합니다. ③ 치실은 치아 사이를 청소하는데 사용합니다.
④ 당신의 이름이 곧 불릴 것이다. ⑤ 립스틱을 휴지로 지웠다.
⑥ 커피나 홍차는 치아를 착색시킬 수 있습니다.

What is plaque?　　　[치면세균막의 성질]

A) Plaque is a sticky film of bacteria that forms on all areas of your teeth.

B) Plaque bacteria can cause cavities and bleeding gums.

C) Plaque is removed by proper brushing, but it will form soon after brushing.

☞ sticky : 끈적끈적한　film : (피)막　bacteria : 세균　form : 형성하다

(A) 치면세균막은 치아에 부착하는 끈적끈적한 세균의 (피)막입니다. (B) 치면세균막의 세균은 충치나 잇몸의 출혈을 일으키는 원인이 됩니다. (C) 치면세균막은 칫솔질을 잘 하면 제거할 수 있지만, 이를 닦은 후 곧 다시 생기기 시작합니다.

What is tartar?　　　[치석의 성질]

A) When plaque isn't removed, it will harden and become tartar.

B) Tartar can lead to gum(periodontal) disease.

C) You can't remove tartar by simple brushing. Tartar can be removed by your dentist or dental hygienist.

☞ when : …때　harden : 단단해지다　become : (…이) 되다　lead : (…결과가) 되다

gum disease : 치주질환(치주병)

A) 치면세균막을 제거하지 않으면 이것이 단단해져 치석이 됩니다. B) 치석은 치주병의 원인입니다.

C) 간단한 칫솔질만으로는 치석을 제거할 수 없습니다. 치석은 치과의사나 치과위생사가 제거합니다.

3. 치아 건강을 위해 당신은 어떻게 하고 계십니까? 양호(○), 불량(×), 보통(△)에 표시를 하고, 그 결과에 대해 토론해 보세요.

① Brush your teeth after eating. (　　　)

② Brush your teeth once a day, after breakfast. (　　　)

③ Brush your teeth once a day, before bedtime. (　　　)

④ Clean between teeth with floss. (　　　)

⑤ Have a balanced diet. (　　　)

⑥ Drink water instead of fruit juices. (　　　)

⑦ Drink some coffee and tea. (　　　)

⑧ Visit your dentist regularly for professional cleanings and examinations. (　　　)

⑨ Eat lots of fruits between meals. (　　　)

☞ ① 식후에 이를 닦는다. ② 하루에 한 번 아침식사 후에 이를 닦는다. ③ 하루에 한 번 잠자기 전에 이를 닦는다. ④ 치실을 사용하여 치아 사이를 닦는다. ⑤ 균형 있는 식사를 한다. ⑥ 과일주스 대신에 물을 마신다. ⑦ 커피나 홍차를 마신다. ⑧ 전문적인 치면세마와 검사를 받기 위해 정기적으로 치과에 간다. ⑨ 식사 중간에 과일을 많이 먹는다.

Answer Key

1

① The clinic is cleaned by us every day.

② I was taken to the station by her.

③ Tartar was removed by the dentist.

④ Your health will be damaged by smoking.

2

② damaged ③ used ④ called ⑤ removed ⑥ caused

UNIT 15 FOCUS

「된다」라는 문장을 만들 때 BE+과거분사를 사용합니다. UNIT 1에서 배운 BE 형태의 사용, UNIT 3에서 배운 현재와 과거의 사용을 복습해 봅시다.

(1) The watch	is	broken.
(2) These watches	are	broken.
(3) Your tooth	was	pulled out.
(4) Your teeth	were	pulled out.

조동사를 사용할 때에는 「뒤의 동사는 그대로」 옵니다. 따라서 수동태일 때에는 BE의 형태는 그대로 be가 됩니다.

(5) My tooth will	be	pulled out.
(6) My tooth should	be	pulled out.
(7) My tooth can	be	pulled out.

Exercise

1. 다음의 문장은 틀린 부분이 있습니다. 잘못된 부분을 찾아 바르게 고치세요.

(1) The window are broken.

(2) The car will is washed by my brother.

(3) Your tooth should be pulled out the dentist.

(4) Our children was injured in the accident.

(5) My finger is cuted.

Exercise

2. 다음 동사의 의미를 사전에서 찾아보세요.

(1) surprise　　(2) excite　　(3) bore

(4) interest　　(5) satisfy

3. 2의 동사는 모두 「~하게 하다」의 뜻이 있습니다. 수동의 형태로 만들면 「~하다」의 의미가 됩니다. 다음의 문장을 영어로 고치세요.

(1) 나는 그 얘기에 놀랐다.

(2) 나는 시합에 흥분할 것이다.

(3) 나는 수업이 지루했다.

(4) 당신은 그 나라에 흥미를 가지게 될지 모릅니다.

(5) 당신은 이 일에 만족해야 합니다.

Answer Key

1

(1) ×are → ○ is

(2) ×is → ○ be　　(3) ×the dentist → ○ by the dentist

(4) ×was → ○ were　　(5) ×cuted → ○ cut

2

(1) surprise: 놀라게 하다　　(2) excite: 흥분하게 하다　　(3) bore: 지루하게 하다

(4) interest: 흥미를 갖게 하다　　(5) satisfy: 만족하게 하다

3

(1) I was surprised at the story.　　(2) I will be excited at the game.

(3) I was bored with the lesson.　　(4) You may be interested in the country.

(5) You should be satisfied with this work.

<역자 약력>

정 원 균(연세대학교 원주의과대학 치위생학과 교수)

정 한 성(연세대학교 치과대학 교수)

김 남 희(연세대학교 원주의과대학 치위생학과 교수)

치과 영어 핸드북

치과종사자를 위한 영어대화의 훈련

발행일 2008년 1월 17일
저 자 Sano Satsuki et al.
역 자 정 원 균 · 정 한 성 · 김 남 희
발행인 최 용 원
편 집 이 은 의
표 지 이 은 의
발행처 **대한나래출판사**
등 록 제2012-000051호(1994.6.10)

주 소 서울특별시 성동구 성수2로 147 (성수동2가 289-319번지)
아이에스비즈타워 903호
전 화 (02) 922-0840
팩 스 (02) 922-0841
이메일 nrpub@naver.com

ISBN 978-89-5741-102-5 **정가 10,000원**